WHAT YOUR
DOCTOR MAY *NOT*
TELL YOU ABOUT™

COLORECTAL
CANCER

WHAT YOUR DOCTOR MAY *NOT* TELL YOU ABOUT™

COLORECTAL CANCER

New Tests, New Treatments,
New Hope

MARK BENNETT POCHAPIN, M.D.

WITH A FOREWORD BY KATIE COURIC

WARNER BOOKS

NEW YORK   BOSTON

The information herein is not intended to replace the services of trained health professionals, or be a substitute for medical advice. You are advised to consult with your health care professional with regard to matters relating to your health, and in particular regarding matters that may require diagnosis or medical attention.

Warner Books

Time Warner Book Group
1271 Avenue of the Americas, New York, NY 10020

Visit our Web site at www.twbookmark.com.

Printed in the United States of America

First Printing: March 2004
10   9   8   7   6   5   4   3   2   1

Library of Congress Cataloging-in-Publication Data
Pochapin, Mark Bennett.
    What your doctor may not tell you about colorectal cancer : new tests, new treatments, new hope / Mark Bennett Pochapin ; with a foreword by Katie Couric.— 1st Warner Books ed.
        p. cm.
    Includes bibliographical references and index.
    ISBN 0-446-53188-X
    1. Colon (Anatomy)—Cancer. 2. Colon (Anatomy)—Cancer—Treatment. 3. Consumer education. I. Title.
RC280.C6P636 2004
616.99'4347—dc22   2003019185

This book is written in loving memory of my mother, **Sandra Pochapin-Kohn,** who passed away after the first manuscript of this book was completed. My mother provided me with what Hodding Carter called "roots" and "wings." "Roots" refers to the family love, values, and traditions that provide the foundation for life. "Wings" are the education, guidance, and support my parents provided that allowed me to "take off" and explore the wonder of creation and experience the joy of a family of my own.

This book is dedicated to my wife, Dr. Shari Midoneck Pochapin, and my two boys, Steven and David Pochapin. Thank you for putting up with my hectic schedule and long hours at work on this book. Shari, you have taught me that together, "for better or for worse," is always better. Steven and David, you have shown me that life's most beautiful word is "Daddy." Thank you all for giving me the gift of your unconditional love. It is my ultimate source of happiness.

Acknowledgments

There are so many people whom I would like to recognize for the roles they played in creating this book and adding to my personal and professional growth. Although the list is quite extensive, there are still so many others *not* on the list who also deserve to be mentioned. However, my editors told me that the acknowledgments couldn't be longer than the text!

To Katie Couric and her associates:

Katie, you have demonstrated that the desire to help others can make a profound positive impact on people's lives, even after suffering such a tragic personal loss. By dedicating yourself to colon cancer awareness, you have saved more lives than any physician. Thank you for your help, dedication, and friendship. May the memory of Jay Monahan live through your children and all the good that you have done for others.

Lisa Paulson, the president/chief executive officer of the Entertainment Industry Foundation and National Colorectal Cancer Research Alliance: Thank you for all your help in creating the Jay Monahan Center and your dedication to raising awareness and funding for cancer education and research.

Kathleen Lobb: Thank you for your endless assistance with every minute detail of the Jay Monahan Center and this book.

To my editors and colleagues who actively participated in the creation of this book:

John Ahern, Lynn Sonberg, and Maggie Robinson were instrumental in the writing, drafting, organization, and production of this book. Thank you for helping me put into words the lifesaving information about colon cancer.

Tamar Wallace, the director of outreach and education at the Jay Monahan Center for Gastrointestinal Health: Thank you for reading every word of the manuscript with interest and purpose to ensure the highest quality and most accurate information.

My office staff, including Nurit Waldman, Annette Ocasio, and Toral Shah: Thank you for keeping me organized and focused, and for allowing my practice to run smoothly.

Dr. Ira Jacobson, the chief of the division of gastroenterology and hepatology at Weill Medical College of Cornell University. Thank you for your leadership and friendship.

The Jay Monahan team of physicians, including Dr. Felice Schnoll-Susman, for help on the hereditary chapters, Dr. Michael Lieberman for reviewing the surgical chapter, Dr. Scott Wadler for his assistance on the oncology chapters, Dr. Lydia Petrovitch for her assistance on the pathology section, and Dr. Sidney Winawer for his comments on the screening recommendations. Thank you for assuring accuracy and completeness.

Rachel Zinamarn, an outstanding cancer nutritionist at Memorial Sloan-Kettering Cancer Center. Thank you for saving the nutrition chapters. Your input, guidance, revisions, and menus were invaluable.

To my family:

My late father, Stuart William Pochapin, taught me the value of human life and the fun of never growing up.

My sister, Margie Bissinger who demonstrates the beauty of having a sister to share in friendship, joy, and sorrow.

My second set of parents, Al and Estelle Midoneck: Thank you for treating me like a son and entrusting to me your beautiful daughter.

My grandparents: Nanny Poe, who taught me the importance of

moments and the power of goodness; Grandma Ruth, who sparked my interest in medicine and always had confidence in me; and Papa Sam, who demonstrated that kindness, gentleness, and a sense of humor are virtues that enrich everyone.

My Aunt Rita and Uncle Phil Rosen showed me by example the importance of family gatherings, giving to charity, and dedicating your life to something you believe in.

My Aunt Shelly and Uncle Ron Goldman have always treated me like a son and showed me how much fun life can be.

To my mentors:

Drs. Joe and Jean Sanger, who were the first to enrich my life with science and give me the opportunity for research at the marine biological laboratory in Woods Hole, Massachusetts.

Dr. Leslie Bernstein, who taught me that regardless of how prestigious your title, no individual is more important than another and that medicine is always filled with wonder.

Dr. Laurence Brandt, who taught me that holding a patient's hand is sometimes more important than examining it.

Dr. Ralph Nachman, the chairman of medicine at Weill Medical College of Cornell, who choose me to be his chief medical resident and showed, by example, how exciting medicine can be from "bench to bedside."

To my patients:

Thank you for entrusting me with the responsibility for your health. You have shown me that no disease can ever eradicate the love for one another or defeat the human spirit—it only strengthens it!

Foreword

My husband Jay was a successful, health-conscious man who watched his diet, exercised regularly, and never smoked. When he was diagnosed with advanced colon cancer at the age of forty-one, we were stunned and devastated.

Before Jay became ill, we had never given colorectal cancer screening a second thought. We didn't know that colorectal cancer is the second leading cancer killer in the United States. We didn't know the fatigue and other vague symptoms Jay felt were signs of colorectal cancer. We didn't know that colorectal cancer is 90 percent curable when found early and, with regular screening, nearly completely preventable.

During Jay's illness, we were fortunate to be under the care of Dr. Mark Pochapin, a highly esteemed gastroenterologist at New York-Presbyterian Hospital/Weill Cornell Medical Center. We learned that colorectal cancer begins with a small noncancerous growth (called a polyp) in the colon or rectum that, over time, can sometimes turn into cancer. Through a simple screening test, polyps can be detected and removed before they become cancerous. Unfortunately, Jay's disease had progressed to an advanced stage by the time it was detected and thus was very difficult to treat.

Mark provided not only the medical expertise of a skilled physician, but also the compassion and caring of a friend, offering guidance and support throughout Jay's diagnosis and treatment. After Jay died, I decided we could and must prevent others from experiencing the loss my family has endured. Why is this preventable disease being allowed to claim the lives of so many men and women, husbands and wives, mothers and fathers, brothers and sisters, friends and loved ones? Why didn't we know about the risk factors and screening tests before it was too late? These were the considerations that prompted me to talk about colorectal cancer screening on NBC's *Today* show, and to co-found the National Colorectal Cancer Research Alliance with Lilly Tartikoff and the Entertainment Industry Foundation. After I had my own colonoscopy on *Today*, I was both surprised and thrilled to learn that colonoscopy screening in the United States increased by nearly 20 percent, according to researchers at the University of Michigan. They decided to call this trend the "Couric Effect"—little did I know I would be associated with colons forevermore! I've been written about in magazines before, but seeing my name in the *Archives of Internal Medicine* was one of the proudest moments of my life.

It is still difficult to fathom that three years after Jay died, I lost my sister Emily—a rising star in the Democratic Party in our home state of Virginia—to pancreatic cancer. Emily's death deepened my resolve to do something more about these insidious and deadly gastrointestinal cancers, including colorectal cancer and pancreatic cancer. As a result, I embarked upon a new collaboration with Mark and his colleagues—the establishment of the Jay Monahan Center for Gastrointestinal Health at NewYork-Presbyterian Hospital/Weill Cornell Medical Center. Under Mark's leadership, the Monahan Center is educating patients and their families, promoting prevention and screening, and providing state-of-the-art treatment and support for those who have or are at risk for a number of gastrointestinal cancers. At the Monahan Center, patients and their families are receiving the best available care, with all health and educational services provided in a way that is seamless and convenient. With Mark at the helm, I know that people seeking information, screening, or treatment at the Monahan Center are in excellent hands.

The even better news is that you do not have to visit the Monahan Center to benefit from Mark's knowledge, dedication, and humanism. This book is a powerful weapon in the fight against colorectal cancer. You can learn how to reduce your risk, recognize the symptoms, and identify the most effective treatment options for colorectal cancer. This book provides the information I wish I had before Jay became ill, and information that can help you and your loved ones deal with this sometimes fatal disease.

Mark is a physician and friend who provided the kind of hand-holding throughout the course of Jay's illness that is often lacking in our medical system. He has also been an invaluable partner in my effort to bring something good from the tragedy of Jay's death. I could not be more pleased that you, too, will have the benefit of Mark's expertise and caring in helping you prevent and fight colorectal cancer.

Before Jay died, he told me something the two of us always knew: "Nothing really matters except your family and friends." I'm sure many of you feel the same way. That's why it's so important that you take care of your health and that your family and friends do the same.

So please, read this book and then see your doctor. It could save your life—or the life of someone you love.

Katie Couric

Contents

Introduction

My beeper startled me as it rang out during dinner. Its piercing sound was a reminder of how doctors like me are forever at the mercy of on-call responsibilities. Responding to the summons of the phone, I headed off to the hospital, as I have done on so many countless nights and weekends. Sometimes life other than medicine has to be put on hold.

I might as well take a moment here to introduce myself. I am a gastroenterologist, a doctor of the colon, stomach, and other parts of the digestive system. For as long as I can remember, I've wanted to be a doctor. Perhaps it was because my Grandma Ruth used to send me cards addressed to "Dr. Mark Pochapin" before I could even speak.

Why I chose gastroenterology is a source of constant amazement to my family and close friends. They know how intensely I dislike odors and discussing bowel habits. What's more, my mother always wanted me to be a plastic surgeon so that I could keep our family looking young!

This entry and exit system in the body—known medically as the gastrointestinal (GI) tract—is one of the most fascinating in all human anatomy, if for no other reason than that it encompasses so many different functions. These include nutrient absorption, enzyme reactions, blood flow, nerve signaling (the body's nerve communication system), hormone control, metabolic reactions, and detoxification. In addition, the gastrointestinal tract is one of the largest immune, or disease-battling, systems in the body. What all this means is that by taking care of the gastrointestinal system and by fostering its ability to work better, doctors and their patients can prevent and fight off disease, including cancers of the colon and rectum (collectively termed colorectal cancer).

It is not an overstatement to say that with a healthy gastrointestinal tract, you will have a healthier body. One of the greatest gifts of life as a doctor is helping people become healthier, and so gastroenterology, with its opportunities to fortify body defenses and perform lifesaving procedures, is a branch of medicine where I felt I could make a real difference.

But back to the story. Among the remarkable things about practicing medicine is that you never know what sort of human drama will unfold with each life you touch. And this night would be no different.

The patient to whose hospital bedside I rushed that evening was a young vital man of forty-one. That he was in the prime of his life, however, was belied by the fact that he was very ill, weak, fatigued, pale, and suffering from terrible abdominal pain. I reviewed a series of tests he had undergone, including blood tests and X rays, and performed an emergency colonoscopy so that I could directly visualize the inside of his colon.

The patient was Jay Monahan, a highly regarded attorney and television legal commentator, the father of two young girls, and the husband of Katie Couric, the popular co-anchor of NBC's *Today* show, whose cheerful countenance warms America's breakfast tables every morning.

I told them that Jay had colorectal cancer—the same grim news that is delivered to approximately 150,000 Americans each year, nearly 60,000 of whom will die from the disease. Sadly, Jay's cancer was found at an advanced stage, and it was invasive, meaning that it had spread well beyond the colon. All the more shocking was that Jay was so young, had no family history of colon cancer, exercised frequently, ate a healthy diet, and never smoked. In other words, Jay had no risk factors for this disease and was the picture of health. Up until this diagnosis, neither Jay nor Katie had ever given colon cancer a second thought. Yet now, because of its intrusion into their lives, what had been an almost fairy-tale existence was shattered.

So began a courageous and, at times, traumatic battle against colon cancer. But it was a battle not to be conquered. Jay died nine months after being diagnosed, two weeks after his forty-second birthday.

Why do I mention all this? Because in the aftermath of Jay's battle, something extraordinary happened.

Until then, the public had not realized how common this killer disease is, nor that screening is available that can save lives and drastically reduce the cases of colorectal cancer each year. It was glaringly evident that one of the most preventable causes of death in this country was swathed in ignorance, misinformation, and an unwillingness on the part of many doctors to recommend lifesaving screening procedures. We so desperately needed better education about colorectal cancer, its risks, and the techniques available to cut those risks.

We were about to get it—not by way of a doctor, a medical researcher, or anyone working in the health care profession. We got it through Katie Couric, who rose from the tragedy and sorrow of her husband's death to launch a national campaign promoting awareness of the importance of screening for colorectal cancer.

In March 2000, Katie Couric, cancer activist Lilly Tartikoff, and the Entertainment Industry Foundation (EIF) co-founded the National Colorectal Cancer Research Alliance (NCCRA). Since then, Katie and the NCCRA have led an initiative to increase public awareness of colorectal cancer and raise millions of research dollars. Important milestones in this effort have included substantial press coverage, with more than four hundred media stories and the *Today* show's broadcast of Katie's own colonoscopy.

The resulting heightened public awareness about colorectal cancer led to an almost 20 percent jump in colonoscopy screening, which University of Michigan researchers dubbed the "Couric Effect." Katie continues to actively promote colorectal cancer awareness on the *Today* show and elsewhere.

Born out of Katie's discussions with me was the Jay Monahan Center for Gastrointestinal Health, a facility dedicated to learning and healing that opened in 2004, where patients can get education, care, treatment, and a little hand-holding for the prevention and treatment of gastrointestinal cancers all coordinated under one roof, without having to run from place to place. So much good had come from so much tragedy.

With the increased attention focused on colorectal cancer, I began to witness the results of the Couric Effect in my own practice, where some of my patients had been stubbornly refusing to get colonoscopies *(You're going to put that* where?*),* no matter how much I pleaded with them. Then all of a sudden, they'd come in and say, "I'm ready to have one." To which I'd respond, "What changed your mind?" Their answer: "I heard Katie talk about it on TV . . ." In fact, one patient even wrote Katie's name on the part of the patient questionnaire that asks: *referred by* _____.

Clearly, one of the biggest problems regarding colorectal cancer is that no one has really wanted to talk about it, perhaps because of embarrassment, or lack of knowledge. With all their time constraints and pressures, doctors, in particular, have been placing it on the back burner, or not talking about it at all. Yet doctors, of all people, need to impress upon their patients the importance of screening and prevention. If doctors aren't talking about it, then their patients won't think it's important, either.

Let's face it: The colon and rectum are not exactly the stuff of watercooler chats or cocktail party conversation. But remaining mum about the subject can cost people their lives. Not that long ago, women felt uneasy discussing breast cancer, and men hardly ever talked about their prostates. Now those cancers are routinely discussed with family, friends, and, most importantly, doctors. We have to do the same for colorectal cancer, because with this disease, what we don't know may hurt us.

I wrote this book to talk openly and forthrightly about colorectal cancer, to continue the forward momentum to conquer this major killer, and, in doing so, to save more lives. I plan to give you the very latest information on colorectal cancer, as well as the best screening and treatment options, in a way that you can understand and use. We know so much more about colorectal cancer than we did just a few years ago. We have a huge array of clinical trials that prove the effectiveness of new drugs and new combinations of drugs. We know that everyday substances, such as calcium and folate, can go a long way toward curbing the disease. In addition we have a wider range of screening and surgical procedures that are lifesaving in their technique and sophistication.

Although words on paper can go only so far, I will provide you with all the resources you need to help prevent this disease, or contend with its potentially devastating presence, should it ever trespass into your life. Think of this book as an opportunity to alter the course of your life and that of your family.

Two of my mentors during my gastroenterology fellowship, Dr. Leslie Bernstein and Dr. Lawrence Brandt, taught me by example the art of being a doctor. I'll never forget Dr. Brandt's platform while serving as president of the American College of Gastroenterology: "Sometimes holding a hand is more important than examining one."

These words echoed what I have always known to be true about practicing medicine, and I adopted them into my own personal philosophy of doctoring. Hand-holding is the ability to connect with patients, listen to them, and respond with compassion, consideration, and respect. It is an important healing component of medicine that, given the current erosion of the doctor–patient relationship, many physicians have forgotten about or don't have time for.

Further, with diseases of the digestive system, there are so many invasive measures taken to diagnose and treat illness that the process can seem undignified, sometimes to the point of sacrificing a person's quality of life. As a doctor, I strive to care about every aspect of my patients' lives while respecting their dignity and privacy. I listen to them, and I encourage them to be fully involved in decisions about their care. And I try to do this in a way that can say more than words—by holding their hand, sometimes physically, but more often in the emotional and figurative sense.

As we go through this book together, learning everything you need to know about colorectal cancer, read it as though I am talking directly to you, but more importantly read it as though I am holding your hand, guiding you at each step along the way.

That said, here's my hand—take it, and let's start talking about what your doctor may not have told you about this disease.

Mark Pochapin, M.D.

Part I

THE DISEASE NO ONE HAS TO DIE FROM

Chapter 1

The Truth About Colorectal Cancer

Life is going to throw you a few curveballs. One day you could suddenly find out that someone you know, someone you love, or perhaps even you, has been diagnosed with cancer of the colon or rectum, referred to together as colorectal cancer. Understandably, you're shocked and confused; if you are the one who is sick, you may simply be unable to absorb the frightening diagnosis. *What does it all mean? How serious is this? Is the dire diagnosis a death sentence? How could this happen to me?*

The frightening truth is that cancer can march unexpectedly into your life, affecting you directly or indirectly by striking someone you love, and colorectal cancer is no different. This year, an estimated 150,000 people in the United States will be diagnosed with colorectal cancer and more than 57,000 of them will die from it. Colorectal cancer is the number two cause of cancer-related deaths among men and women combined. These statistics are a grim reminder of a fact that most people would rather ignore: Cancers of the colon and rectum are relatively common—and can be deadly.

But the good news—no, the *great* news—is that when found in its earliest stage, colorectal cancer can be cured fully more than 90 percent of the time! That said, I wish the story concluded there, but unhappily, we rarely find cancer in this early, curable stage, because not enough people are being screened for it.

A survey from the *Harvard Report on Cancer Prevention* shows that as many as 80 percent of Americans are not following the proper screening recommendations. Admittedly, many people shrink from the idea of colorectal cancer screening tests such as a colonoscopy because they are afraid of the preparation and procedure. More alarmingly, many health care practitioners simply are not telling their patients to get the recommended tests! Too few people understand that failing to undergo these tests means missing the chance to have potentially precancerous growths called *polyps* removed and facing a poor long-term outcome in the event that cancer is found in its later stages.

Colorectal cancer is in part a genetic disease, but one that is influenced greatly by your lifestyle—what you eat, whether you smoke, how active you are, how often you undergo routine screening, and, in general, how you live your life, day in and day out—all issues I will discuss in this book. As doctors, we now believe that, despite the role of genetics, almost all colorectal cancers can be prevented through lifestyle changes *and* regular screening. Just think: You can beat this disease with the right medical decisions and positive living.

A JOURNEY THROUGH YOUR DIGESTIVE SYSTEM

So that you can better understand the nature of colorectal cancer and how it affects your body, an important first step is to learn more about the fascinating inner workings of your digestive system. I'll run through an anatomy lesson with you, explaining key processes up front so that you can get comfortable with the terms I will be using throughout the book. For starters, let's follow a meal—say, a tuna salad sandwich—as it winds its way from your mouth down the twenty-five-foot tunnel commonly known as your digestive tract.

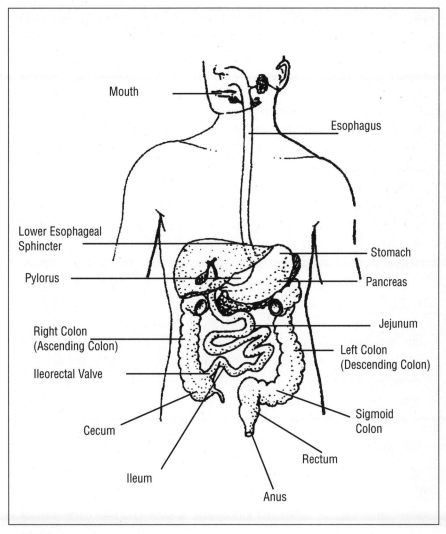

Mouth

Esophagus

Lower Esophageal Sphincter

Stomach

Pylorus

Pancreas

Jejunum

Right Colon (Ascending Colon)

Left Colon (Descending Colon)

Ileorectal Valve

Sigmoid Colon

Cecum

Rectum

Ileum

Anus

FIGURE 1

The Mouth

That sandwich you've just had for lunch begins its digestion in your mouth, where it is chewed and broken down by chemicals (enzymes) in your saliva into more absorbable forms. The carbohydrate in the bread, the protein in the tuna, and the fat in the mayonnaise each has its own set of digestive enzymes that go to work at various stages of digestion. An enzyme in your saliva, for example, begins the digestion of carbohydrates into simple sugars.

The Esophagus

Once a few bites of your sandwich have been chewed, moistened, and broken down, you swallow it—a process that involves many muscles working in sync to move the food down your esophagus (food pipe) into your stomach.

When your food arrives at the lower end of the esophagus, there is a valve, one of many "gates" that open and close, controlling entry to each digestive organ along the way. These valves are called sphincters. They keep food and other material from passing backward into places where they shouldn't go.

Beginning in the esophagus, food moves smoothly through your entire digestive tract via a process called peristalsis, a coordinated, rhythmic wave of muscular contraction that travels in a single direction. Peristalsis works independently of gravity. You could eat while standing on your head, for instance, and food would still move from your esophagus to your stomach and through your system.

The Stomach

Your stomach stores the food material for hours and starts churning it into a more liquid form called chyme. Enzymes continue their work of breaking down the tuna salad sandwich. The digestion of protein occurs in your stomach, with proteins being chopped into microscopic fragments called amino acids. Protein can also be digested elsewhere in the digestive system, so even if you had your entire stomach removed, you could still digest food.

Another interesting aspect of the stomach is its production of hydrochloric acid. This acid is so corrosive that it can eat its way through metal. Fortunately, the inner lining of your stomach has a protective layer of mucus, or the acid would burn right through your stomach wall. Sometimes, acid can cause diseases such as ulcers and gastroesophageal reflux disease (GERD), but these are treatable with medications designed to block excessive acid production.

Hydrochloric acid is there for a reason: It activates some digestive enzymes in the stomach and it sterilizes the food you eat. Sterilizing food may not be such a big deal today because the food we eat is fairly clean and often cooked. It was a huge advantage ages ago, however, when early humans ingested bug-infested tree bark and rotting dead animals. Thank goodness for the invention of refrigeration and the supermarket! If you are taking medications to reduce stomach acid, don't worry. Our food supply is so clean and the digestion of nutrients is so repetitive in the gastrointestinal system that even complete acid suppression is well tolerated by the body.

But back to that tuna salad sandwich: In its now partially digested form, it will usually sit in your stomach for two to four hours.

The Small Intestine

Your stomach empties the now liquefied sandwich into your small intestine via a sphincter known as the pyloric valve, which prevents the passage of partially digested food until it has been properly processed by your stomach. Made up of three segments—the duodenum, jejunum, and ileum—your small intestine is roughly twenty-one feet in length and coiled loosely in the part of your body commonly called the abdomen. When my patients tell me that they feel food and gas moving in their "stomach," what they are usually sensing is the movement of their small intestine as it digests food.

In the small intestine, food is further broken down, and the jejunum and ileum are primarily responsible for absorbing the nutrients so they can be used to support the health and energy needs of your body. The lining of your small intestine is filled with closely packed, fingerlike projections called villi that greatly increase the amount of surface area available for absorbing nutrients. If all of these villi were spread out flat, their surface area would span the length of a tennis court, or about two hundred square feet. Incidentally, cancer is extremely rare in the small intestine.

Other Digestive Organs

Other digestive organs are involved in digestion. One is your pancreas, a flask-shaped organ situated just behind your stomach, toward the back. Its job is to secrete digestive enzymes into the small intestine in order to break down protein, carbohydrates, and fats. Apart from its digestive function, your pancreas also produces two hormones, insulin and glucagon, that are released into the blood and together help regulate the normal rise and fall in blood sugar.

All the absorbed nutrients from digestion eventually pass through your liver, the largest solid organ in your body. The carbohydrate from the bread of the tuna sandwich, for example, arrives there as simple sugars. The liver converts these sugars to glucose, your body's primary fuel. Any glucose not used for fuel is stored in your liver or in your muscles as a larger molecule known as glycogen. The liver can also turn protein and fat into glucose if your body requires additional energy sources.

Among its many other functions, your liver also manufactures and secretes bile. Bile is a greenish liquid containing bile salts that emulsify, or break up, dietary fat so that it can be further broken down by enzymes.

Situated just under the liver is a pear-shaped organ known as the gallbladder. Its job is to receive bile from the liver and store it. During a meal, your gallbladder contracts and squirts bile into your duodenum through a tube called the common bile duct.

The Colon

Once the nutrients have been absorbed by your small intestine and processed by your liver, what is left of that tuna salad sandwich moves on by peristalsis to your colon, a muscular tube between four and six feet in length. The colon connects your small intestine to the rectum, the last part of the digestive tract. By the time the sandwich reaches your colon, the remaining material consists of undigested food particles (such as fiber), water, and secretions from your small intestine.

At the origin of the colon is a small pouch named the cecum, which includes an opening into a tiny nonfunctional tube called the appendix. This region is located in the lower right part of the abdomen and is also the site where the small intestine joins the colon. Anatomically, the colon is made up of four sections: the ascending (right) colon; the transverse (across) colon, which hangs like a necklace down to as low as your belly button; the descending (left) colon, which moves down the left side toward your pelvic area; and the sigmoid colon (so named for its S shape, derived from the Greek letter *S*, sigma). Cancer can develop in any of these four sections, as well as in your rectum.

Your colon is constructed of four layers of tissue. The innermost layer, the mucosa, is smooth, thin, and has no villi. It has direct contact with the material that passes through the colon. The cells of the mucosa are in a constant state of replenishment, dying, sloughing off, and being replaced by new cells about every four to six days. Underneath the mucosa is the submucosa, a layer of tissue that provides support for the mucosa. The submucosa also harbors the white blood cells (lymphocytes, monocytes, and neutrophils) that keep bacteria from the colon out of the bloodstream. The third layer is the muscularis propria, made up of muscle cells that assist in movement. Finally, the fourth and outermost layer is the serosa, which provides added strength to the colon and serves as a protective barrier.

Sometimes the term *colon* is used interchangeably with *large intestine*. I dislike using the term *large intestine* because the small intestine is actually much longer than the colon. Therefore, so as not to confuse matters, I will use the term *colon* rather than *large intestine,* although these terms do refer to the same organ. The term *bowel* generally refers to any part of the intestine, large or small.

The primary duties of the colon are to absorb water and electrolytes, such as sodium and potassium, from the intestinal material and to compact solid waste so that it can be eliminated from your body. Think of the colon as a large "dryer" removing the water from the wet material left by the small intestine. As water is extracted in the colon, the material becomes more solid. In this state, it is called stool or feces. Stool moves upward from the cecum into the ascending colon, across the abdomen in the transverse colon, and then down the left side of your abdomen in the descending and sigmoid colons, where it is stored until being emptied into the rectum, usually once or twice a day.

Your colon also harbors an enormous colony of bacteria. When you hear about bacteria, it often brings to mind all those TV commercials showing us how to rid ourselves and our environment of these nasty bugs. Cleanliness seems to be forever equated with being germ-free. This is not an accurate depiction, however. There are, of course, pathogenic (disease-causing) bacteria in our environment, but most of the bacteria that we encounter are friendly and actually assist in the functioning of our digestion. Scientists theorize that the energy factory within our cells (the mitochondria) were at one time bacteria that joined our cells during an evolutionary process to form a mutually beneficial relationship. The reasoning behind this theory is that mitochondria have a DNA that is more similar to bacteria than it is to human DNA. So bacteria shouldn't always be stereotyped as being the bad guys; many are our friends.

Here is another interesting fact: By numbers alone, there are more bacteria in and on each of us than there are human cells in our bodies. In some ways, we are more bacteria than human!

The helpful bacteria in the body, known as the normal flora, promote health and immunity in a variety of ways. First of all, they help stimulate the immune system's production of disease-fighting white blood cells. Second, they form a protective barrier in order to keep levels of bad bacteria from attaching to the colon walls and being absorbed. Third, they produce certain types of acid that discourage harmful organisms such as yeast from proliferating. Fourth, some normal flora synthesize certain B vitamins for proper metabolism, as well as vitamin K, which is essential to normal blood clotting. Finally, these bacteria help change fecal matter into a form that can be properly eliminated.

The presence of these friendly bacteria makes your colon an important organ of immunity. There is a vast interplay between the white blood cells in the intestine and the normal flora. Without these health-promoting bacteria in your colon, your body is less capable of functioning normally and fighting off disease.

As a whole, the digestive tract is the largest immune organ inside your body. Think about it. When we eat, we ingest foreign material that is loaded with environmental bacteria. The small intestines have to keep the bacteria out of the body, while absorbing the nutrients. Moreover, the intestines must decide if the ingested bacteria is safe or disease producing. As we discuss the specifics of colorectal cancer later in this book, the concept of the digestive tract, specifically the small intestine and colon, as an immune organ becomes important.

The Rectum

Although most people are usually too embarrassed to talk about the rectum, it is actually a vital part of the gastrointestinal tract—really. You may have heard a story about a debate among the body's organs as to which was the most important. When the rectum boldly asserted its importance, other organs like the brain and heart responded with derisive laughter. The rectum became so upset that it decided to shut down for a while and show the other body parts just how important it was. So the rectum closed up shop, and it wasn't long before the brain became foggy, the heart started beating faster, and the stomach felt queasy. Finally they all couldn't take it any longer and declared unanimously that the rectum was the most important part of the body.

If you have ever experienced a "work stoppage" of your rectum, you'll appreciate the truth of this story. There can be a great deal of abdominal discomfort and cramping if your rectum is not performing its job of storing and evacuating stool from your colon.

Understanding the anatomy of both the colon and rectum is essential because colorectal cancer can occur in any part of these two organs. Further, the location of the disease plays a role in the type of treatment that is required.

The Anus

The rectum works in concert with the anus, located at the very end of the digestive tract. There, anal sphincter muscles block the movement of stool and prevent it from coming out when it is not supposed to. Together, the rectum and the anus expel stool. The pressure of the stool in the rectum stimulates movement. As a result, the rectal muscles contract, and the anal sphincter relaxes. Provided you're ready and in a bathroom, the anal sphincter relaxes under voluntary control and the stool is pushed out of your body. If you must "hold it" when the urge occurs, the anus remains closed until you can find a bathroom.

The time it takes for that tuna salad sandwich to enter at the mouth and exit at the anus is called transit time. If you eat a healthy diet, with plenty of water and fiber, your transit time should be just over a day.

THE FIVE DEADLIEST MYTHS ABOUT COLORECTAL CANCER

Now that you have a basic understanding of how your gastrointestinal tract works when it's healthy, I'd like to take our journey a step further by explaining some common myths about colorectal cancer. Don't let these myths get in your way of having regular screening tests and taking other measures to prevent colorectal cancer.

Myth 1: Only Old People Get It; Young People Don't

Here we start with a myth that is scary in its ramifications.

Statistically, the incidence of colorectal cancer does begin to rise sharply as you get older, but even young adults in their twenties can get colorectal cancer. It is estimated that nearly 7 percent of colorectal cancer cases occur in people younger than age fifty. Consider the story of Molly McMaster, an ice-skating teacher and hockey coach in Colorado who was diagnosed with colon cancer in 1999 after enduring months of constipation and abdominal pain that resulted in so many days off from work that she was fired from her job. Molly headed to her hometown of Glenn Falls, New York, where she had emergency surgery that removed the cancer and twenty-five inches of her colon. Determined to create meaning out of her experience, Molly skated across the country, from Glenn Falls to Greeley, Colorado, a seventy-one-day, two-thousand-mile trip that ended in July 2000 in order to raise money and awareness for colorectal cancer. Molly's most recent educational creation is an amazing forty-foot crawl-through "Colossal Colon" that has been touring the United States. When the Colossal Colon came to visit New York City, I had the privilege of working with Molly and the Cancer Research and Prevention Foundation, and let me tell you, this lovely young vibrant woman is certainly not the person you would expect to have colon cancer. You see, when Molly was diagnosed with this disease, she was only twenty-three years old.

The story of Jay Monahan I shared with you in the Introduction should be another loud wake-up call that colorectal cancer does indeed strike the young. And it can strike a second time. Young people who have already had colorectal cancer, particularly those younger then forty, have a higher risk for getting colorectal cancer a second time than do people in older age groups. So please don't kid yourself. Although it does occur more frequently in people fifty and older, younger people can also succumb to colorectal cancer. And as you will hear me say again and again throughout this book: Caught in its earliest stages, colorectal cancer is curable more than 90 percent of the time.

Myth 2: Colorectal Cancer Is a Man's Disease

Don't ever believe this, not for one second! Although certain diseases occur more frequently in men than in women (or vice versa) colorectal cancer is not one of them. The truth of the matter is that colorectal cancer is an equal opportunity disease, striking both men and women with similar frequency.

For my women readers: Believing that colorectal cancer is a man's disease can be dangerous. Please be as aware of colorecal cancer as you are of breast or cervical cancer—add colorectal cancer screening to your list of must-have tests, right there with your mammogram and Pap test.

Myth 3: No One in My Family Ever Had Colorectal Cancer, so I'm Not at Risk

So many people believe this myth that it is sad, really sad. It is true that people with a strong family history of colorectal cancer are at increased risk for this disease. However, please understand that for nearly 80 percent of all people who get colorectal cancer, the disease does *not* run in the family. But let's forget statistics for a moment and talk about real life. In my fifteen years of practicing medicine, I have seen far too many patients with no family history of the disease who sadly found themselves with invasive colorectal cancer. Truthfully, most of these people never had a screening test. They believed they just didn't need it or were never told about it because colorectal cancer didn't run in their family. I say this not to point a finger, but instead to hold your hand and reassure you that this disease is highly treatable and highly curable when caught in its earliest stages.

Myth 4: I Don't Need to Worry About Colorectal Cancer, I Feel Fine

This is the worst myth of them all. What do you think is the most common symptom of early colorectal cancer? Did you say blood in the stool or perhaps constipation? Well, this is actually a trick question because there are often no symptoms at all. People who have early colorectal cancer feel just fine. Only when the cancer grows does it cause symptoms. We believe that in average-risk individuals all colorectal cancers begin as a polyp that transforms over the course of years into cancer. Early on, when the cancer is small, it is painless and symptom free. The good news is that when a symptom-free person gets screened, even the worst scenario of finding a small cancer frequently results in a cure. The bottom line is not to wait for symptoms, but to get screened when you are feeling well.

Myth 5: Colorectal Cancer Always Starts with Blood in the Stool

This myth is based in some reality but it is dangerous because the sight of rectal blood often causes immediate fear. Most of the time, rectal bleeding is caused by hemorrhoidal swelling and inflammation. Yes, colorectal cancers can bleed, however, the amount of blood lost in the stool may be microscopic and not visible to the naked eye. In fact, bleeding may not occur at all. However, if a cancer or large polyp does bleed, this *could* appear as blood in the stool. Frequently, the bleeding can be so subtle that the only symptom is fatigue from mild iron deficiency anemia (low blood count). Anemia can only be detected by a blood test known as a complete blood count (CBC) that determines the amount of red blood cells (hemoglobin and hematocrit values).

Blood in the stool is only one of the many symptoms that larger colorectal cancers can create. Remember, the earliest and smallest colorectal cancers are completely silent (see myth 4). Larger cancers can cause the signs and symptoms listed in the sidebar below. The changes in bowel habits occur because the cancer begins to narrow the inside of the colon, making it difficult for stool to pass. This is the reason a person may develop constipation, bloating, cramping, thinner or looser stool, or incomplete evacuation. In more advanced colorectal cancer, loss of appetite and/or unexplained weight loss can be noticed. These symptoms may occur from chemicals released by the cancer into the bloodstream as it grows and spreads (metastasizes) throughout the body. So, if you have any of the signs or symptoms of colorectal cancer listed below, it is very important that you see a doctor.

Don't let any of these myths stand in the way of possibly saving your life someday. Please don't.

Checklist of Signs and Symptoms of Colorectal Cancer

If you're like most people, you may be uncomfortable talking about your intestinal functions. You've got to change your thinking. If you're not the one to tell your doctor about unusual symptoms—such as your stools changing shape—he or she will never know and sometimes may not even ask! Here's an overview of what to look for.

Don't get frightened. Most of these symptoms are common and unrelated to cancer. However, let your doctor be the judge, not you:

- Change in bowel habits, including new and persistent loose stools; new or unusual constipation; uncomfortable bowel movements; pencil-thin stools; stools that appear more narrow than usual; and the feeling of incomplete emptying of the bowels.

- New abdominal discomfort such as gas, pain, bloating, cramping, or fullness.

- Bleeding (bright red or very dark blood in the stool).

- Constant fatigue.

- Unexplained weight loss.

- Unexplained iron deficiency.

- Unexplained anemia.

Chapter 2

Risk Factors:
Who Gets Colorectal Cancer and Why?

How in the world does colorectal cancer start in the first place? This is a question that I'm frequently asked by my patients, and I know it's on your mind, too. Let's begin to answer it by looking at how colorectal cancer starts and who is at risk.

Cancer, in general, is a disease characterized by out-of-control cell growth and division. Under normal conditions, the cells in your body continually reproduce themselves, with newer cells being formed and older cells naturally dying out. This process of orderly and planned cell death is called *apoptosis*. When it works as it should, your body maintains a balance of new and old cells, and you stay healthy.

Governing the process of apoptosis are genes found in the nucleus of every cell and constructed of strands of DNA (deoxyribonucleic acid), which dictate instructions on everything from your eye color to your height. Genes also produce proteins that issue signals to cells, telling them when to grow, divide, or die out.

Cancer can develop when a number of these genes suffer permanent damage (called a mutation) in a single cell over a lifetime. Mutations can be the result of hereditary factors, lifestyle offenders such as smoking or diet, or a combination of the two.

When mutated, genes begin to act abnormally. They overproduce growth-stimulating proteins, or, in some cases, their ability to suppress tumor growth gets turned off. As a result, the process of apoptosis to suppress tumor growth gets turned off and cells don't self-destruct as they normally should. These abnormal cells start to divide at a rapid rate, eventually forming a cancerous growth. This rapid division continues, and the cancer grows and spreads well beyond the spot where it originally started. This process is known as metastasis.

GENES AND COLORECTAL CANCER

Among the genes involved in colorectal cancer are:

• **APC and P53 tumor suppressor genes:** Normally, these genes turn off the process of cell division and are responsible for halting the formation of tumors by controlling the rate of cell division. Losing or damaging a tumor suppressor gene is often compared to losing the brakes in your car: When this gene is faulty, there is uncontrolled, runaway cell growth, like a car that is careening out of control.

• **RAS oncogene:** Ordinarily, oncogenes and tumor suppressor genes work together to regulate normal cell division. While tumor suppressor genes are responsible for switching off the process of cell growth, oncogenes turn it on. But when an oncogene gets damaged by mutation, or accidentally gets duplicated during cell division, it can trigger rampant cell division that leads to cancer. Whereas a mutated tumor suppressor gene is like a car with no brakes, a mutated oncogene is often compared to a car where the accelerator is stuck to the floorboard. It just keeps on producing more and more cells, and the process of abnormal cell division speeds up.

• **hMSH2 and hMLH1 genes:** These genes signal proteins responsible for DNA repair so that mistakes made during cell reproduction can be corrected. Mutations in these genes interfere with this repair process and are believed to allow errors to accumulate in other key genes that regulate cell growth.

THE POLYP-TO-CANCER SEQUENCE

Most cancers of the colon or rectum are thought to begin as benign *polyps,* a term that first came into our national consciousness in the 1980s when then president Ronald Reagan was diagnosed with colon cancer. A positive fecal occult blood test (FOBT) led to the finding of polyps, one of which was cancerous. Polyps are round growths protruding from the inner lining of the colon or rectum. They may be flat, or they may resemble a stalk of broccoli with beadlike projections.

Although most polyps remain benign, some may grow and transform into cancerous (malignant) tumors if they are not removed. The process whereby a polyp turns cancerous is most likely caused by a series of genetic mutations in the cells. There are a few different types of polyps, but the only type believed to be capable of turning cancerous is referred to as an *adenomatous polyp.*

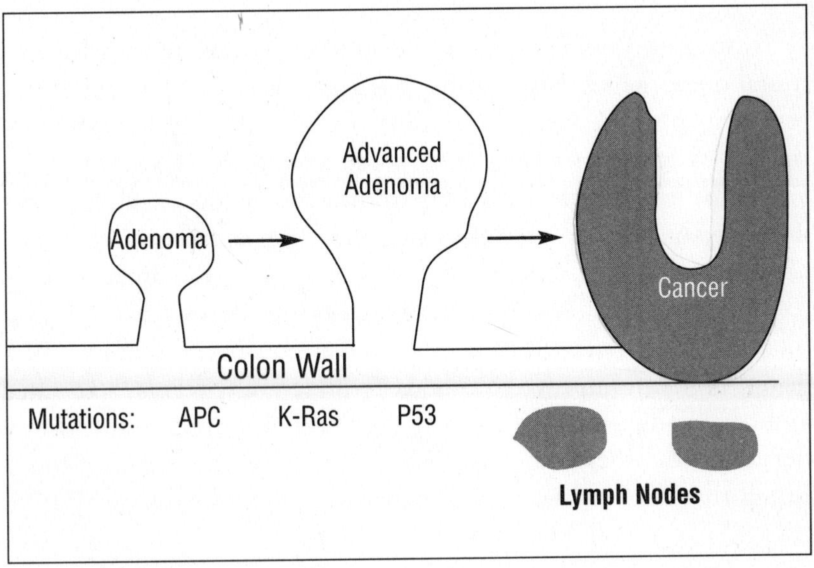

FIGURE 2

Unless you undergo medical screening with a procedure such as a colonoscopy, you'll never know for sure whether a polyp is growing inside your colon or rectum, because there are usually no symptoms. Large polyps or cancer, however, can cause bleeding, microscopic blood in the stool, anemia, or even blockage of the colon. These symptoms are rare and develop only when the polyp becomes quite sizable or malignant.

Colorectal cancer does not develop overnight; it is estimated to take five to fifteen years for an adenomatous polyp to become cancerous. If an adenomatous polyp goes undetected for many years, it may turn into a malignant tumor. As the tumor grows, it can burrow more deeply into the wall of the colon or rectum, eventually invading nearby organs. Should colorectal cancer enter the lymph nodes or bloodstream, it can spread, or metastasize, to other parts of the body, such as the liver, lungs, or brain. At that stage of progression, it becomes much more challenging to treat colorectal cancer.

To sum up: Nearly all cancers of the colon and rectum involve mutations in genes. Many of the mutations leading up to colorectal cancer involve the loss or disabling of genes that suppress the formation of tumors or keep normal cell growth in check. The prevailing belief, though, is that environmental factors, while they do not directly cause colorectal cancer, may trigger the genetic mutations that lead to it. Put another way, genes are like a light waiting to be switched on; environmental factors are the switch that turns on, or activates, those genes. But even if you have inherited "bad genes," you can improve your odds by undergoing regular screening and developing healthy lifestyle habits. Thus, it's important to understand your personal risk factors for colorectal cancer—those things that raise or lower your chance of getting the disease.

ARE YOU AT RISK?

With colorectal cancer, as with other serious diseases, identifying red-flag medical conditions, along with glitches in your diet and lifestyle, could signal the need for earlier and perhaps more frequent medical screening, treatment, or sweeping changes in your day-to-day habits. In other words, knowing your risk factors could save your life.

You may feel healthy, energetic, doing everything right in your life. You're not even thinking about colorectal cancer. But are you at increased risk or not? Here is a look at the specific factors—which include age, family medical history, personal medical history, and lifestyle factors—that influence your odds of developing colorectal cancer.

Increasing Age

For most people today, age is the largest risk factor for colorectal cancer. Although colorectal cancer can affect young people, the disease strikes primarily people age fifty and older. In fact, nearly 90 percent of all colorectal cancer is found in people over fifty.

Why is age such a significant risk factor? The chief reason is that it takes many years for cellular and genetic changes to take place in the lining of the colon or rectum in order for polyps to develop. The older you get, the more likely you are to have polyps. At age fifty, about 10 percent of all Americans have polyps, and by age seventy, nearly 30 percent will have them. If left untreated, a small percentage of these polyps can turn malignant. The only way to know whether a polyp is cancerous is to find it, remove it, and have it evaluated under a microscope.

Hereditary Colorectal Cancer

Approximately 75 to 80 percent of all colorectal cancer occurs in people without a family history of the disease. But in the remaining 20 to 25 percent, susceptibility can be passed down from generation to generation, just like blue eyes or a dimpled chin. In an even smaller percentage of cases (around 5 percent), a patient may have inherited a genetic abnormality that *causes* colorectal cancer. One such abnormality is termed hereditary nonpolyposis colorectal cancer (HNPCC), and the other is familial adenomatous polyposis (FAP). Although these inherited conditions are rare, they can be deadly if not detected, diagnosed, and treated early. Moreover, these diseases can teach us important information about the genetics of colorectal cancer—information that benefits everyone.

HEREDITARY NONPOLYPOSIS COLORECTAL CANCER (HNPCC)

The most common inherited form of colorectal cancer is hereditary nonpolyposis colorectal cancer, and it accounts for less than 5 percent of all cases. The name is somewhat confusing because it contains the term *nonpolyposis* (meaning "no polyp"), even though the cancer still arises from a polyp. What *nonpolyposis* really means, however, is that there are not thousands of polyps as there are in the other hereditary condition known as FAP.

First identified in 1966, HNPCC is caused by mutations in several genes, including hMSH2 and hMLH1, which are responsible for repairing errors in your DNA. Each time a cell divides, it makes a duplicate copy of its DNA, although sometimes mistakes occur and the copy isn't exact. Under normal circumstances, special DNA repair enzymes identify and correct these defective copies, working much like a molecular spell-checker to fix errors. But when DNA repair genes are mutated—a condition known as microsatellite instability (MSI)—the copies aren't fixed, mutations pile up, and the risk of cancer growth increases. Although MSI is a hallmark of HNPCC, it is also present in approximately 15 percent of non-HNPCC-related colorectal tumors.

In HNPCC, potentially cancerous polyps begin to form before the age of twenty, and most of these polyps develop in the right side of the colon. On average, if colorectal cancer is to develop, a person with HNPCC may get full-blown cancer at around age forty-five, whereas someone without hereditary risk factors may get cancer at around age sixty-three.

Patients and family members with HNPCC are also at risk for a wide variety of other cancers, including cancers of the endometrium or uterus, ovary, bile duct, pancreas, stomach, small intestine, brain, and urinary tract. These other cancers are important to recognize as sometimes being genetically linked to colorectal cancer. If a close family member is diagnosed at a young age with any of these other malignancies, this may represent a possible red flag that the family is at increased risk for colorectal cancer and needs to begin screening between the ages of twenty and thirty.

HNPCC-Related Cancers

- Endometrial (uterine) cancer.
- Ovarian cancer.
- Stomach cancer.
- Hepatobiliary cancer. This is a cancer that occurs on or in the liver, bile ducts, and biliary tract—the tubes that carry bile from the liver or gallbladder to the small intestine.
- Small intestine cancer.
- Cancers of the kidney and urinary tract—specifically, transitional cell carcinoma, which starts in the renal pelvis, where the ureter and kidney meet.
- Pancreatic cancer.
- Brain cancer.

HNPCC is diagnosed primarily on family history, using certain family-profile characteristics known as the modified Amsterdam II criteria. Think of these criteria as the rule of 3-2-1:

- At least *three* of your relatives had colorectal cancer (or associated cancers), and one of these relatives is a first-degree relative of the other two.
- *Two* successive generations are involved.
- *One* or more of these family members was diagnosed with colorectal cancer (or associated cancers) prior to age fifty.

If any hereditary or familial cancer syndrome is suspected when colorectal cancer is discovered (even if the HNPCC rule of 3-2-1 does not apply), I believe it is very important for the tumor to be evaluated for MSI. Testing colorectal cancer for MSI is relatively new and your doctor may not know about it. However, if the tumor harbors MSI, then the individual with colorectal cancer should be tested to locate the exact genetic defect. If this defect is isolated, then all family members can be tested for it, too. Diagnosing HNPCC in a family may have a profound lifesaving effect on young family members who otherwise may not know to start screening for colorectal cancer as early as ages twenty to twenty-five (see table 2-2).

FAMILIAL ADENOMATOUS POLYPOSIS (FAP)

This syndrome is caused by a mutation of the adenomatous poly-posis coli (APC) gene, normally responsible for tumor suppression. In FAP, hundreds to thousands of benign polyps form in the colon, beginning as early as the teen years, and eventually one will always turn malignant. Fortunately, FAP is extremely rare. If one of your parents has this disease, then you have a 50 percent chance of in-heriting the gene (this is known as autosomal dominant). About half the people with this syndrome will develop polyps in their teenage years; and 95 percent, by age thirty-five. Everyone with FAP will develop colon cancer, usually by the age of forty, unless they have their colon surgically removed to prevent the disease. Genetic testing (see below) can identify the presence of defective genes in both FAP and HNPCC.

GENETIC TESTING FOR FAP AND HNPCC

Specific genetic tests are now available for people considered at high risk for inherited colorectal cancer. The cost of these genetic tests ranges from $300 to $2,000, and now many insurance carriers cover the cost. Should you test positive for any of these mutations, you will need a colonoscopy and other screening tests as recom-mended by your doctor at regular intervals in order to detect pre-cancerous changes in your colon and rectum. See the screening guidelines in chapters 3 and 4 for information on how frequently you should be getting tested according to your risk level.

An important part of genetic testing is genetic counseling, which involves face-to-face counseling with a professional genetic coun-selor or hereditary cancer-specialist. During these sessions, you will be asked to compile a detailed personal and family medical history that:

- Includes three generations.
- Identifies cancer of all types occurring in relatives.
- Records the family member's age when he or she was diagnosed with cancer.
- Documents and reviews available test reports (yours and your relatives').

Counseling should also cover the medical aspects of the genetic disorder, provide information about the genetic tests available, and review recommended screening guidelines. Your doctor should be able to refer you to the appropriate genetic counselor for help.

Ashkenazi Jewish Descent

About 6 percent of the Jewish population with relatives from Eastern Europe (Ashkenazi Jews) has double the risk of developing colorectal cancer. These patients carry a mutation in the APC tumor suppressor gene. This mutation, however, does not lead to FAP, but instead causes a second error that interrupts the normal function of the APC gene, increasing the odds of colon or rectal cancer. Individuals of Ashkenazi Jewish descent with any family history of colorectal cancer should speak to their doctors about early screening.

African Americans at Higher Risk

African American men and women need to be especially tuned into regular screenings for colorectal cancer. This is because current data show that African Americans who develop colorectal cancer are more likely to die from the disease than their Caucasian counterparts. In addition, compared to Caucasians, African Americans are more likely to develop polyps much deeper in the colon in the right, or ascending, colon. This part of the colon is not visualized by a flexible sigmoidoscopy examination. Since a colonoscopy views the entire colon, including the right side, I particularly encourage my

African American patients to have a colonoscopy rather than a flexible sigmoidoscopy.

From 1992 to 1998, the five-year survival rate for African Americans was 10 percent below that of Caucasians. This discrepancy in survival may be due in part to African Americans being diagnosed with more advanced disease, perhaps related to the increased number of right-sided colon polyps. But there may also be some differences between African Americans and Caucasians in the treatment or care they receive. I urge my African American readers to take the initiative and ask your doctor about reducing your risk and being screened for colorectal cancer, preferably with a colonoscopy. Remember, if you catch this cancer before it starts, you can prevent it altogether.

Your Family History

Apart from the specific inherited colorectal cancer syndromes, you run a greater risk for getting colorectal cancer if you have a strong family history of either colorectal cancer or adenomatous polyps. This is particularly true if a first-degree relative (parent, sibling, or child) had colorectal cancer or adenomatous polyps before age fifty. However, a history of colorectal cancer in distant relatives can increase your risk as well.

In addition to colorectal cancer and polyps, there is some evidence that a family history of certain related cancers—such as endometrial (uterine), stomach, and ovarian cancers—may place you at increased risk for colorectal cancer. While these related cancers are not included in the formal recommended colorectal cancer screening guidelines, I would urge you to discuss any family history of these cancers with your doctor.

My recommendation? Make a list of all your family members for three generations, find out about all cancers and polyps, and share this information with your doctor. Knowing your family history may give your doctor reason to start screening for colorectal cancer *early* (before age fifty).

Your Personal Medical History

A variety of medical conditions can increase your chances of developing colorectal cancer. One serious risk factor is having had colorectal cancer previously. Even if you were cured of colorectal cancer, your risk of developing a new colon or rectum cancer is higher than that of someone at average risk. Similarly, having had recurrent adenomatous polyps also elevates your risk for colorectal cancer, particularly if the polyps were large and numerous. Other types of polyps, such as hyperplastic polyps, are not generally considered to be a risk factor for colorectal cancer.

Another factor that confers a greater risk is a personal history of inflammatory bowel disease, namely ulcerative colitis or Crohn's disease. These bowel diseases cause inflammation, tiny ulcers, and small abscesses in the inner lining of your intestine. While Crohn's disease may affect the small intestine or colon (or both), ulcerative colitis generally affects only the colon and rectum. If you have suffered from severe inflammatory bowel disease over the years, your risk of developing colorectal cancer is significantly greater than that of the general population. One possible explanation for this increased risk is that the cells in the colon grow and divide too rapidly. Consequently, the cells have less time to repair DNA damage, and DNA damage can lead to colorectal cancer.

In addition to these risk factors, there is some evidence that a personal history of certain related cancers—such as endometrial (uterine), stomach, and ovarian cancers—may place you at increased risk for colorectal cancer. Emerging research also suggests a possible increased risk of colorectal cancer in women who have had breast cancer. These other cancers may not appear in any of the formal recommended screening guidelines (see tables 4-1A,B), but can be important to help your doctor decide when to start colorectal cancer screening.

As with your family medical history, I would encourage you to make a list of your personal medical history and share this information with your doctor. It is information that could help to save your life.

YOUR HABITS AND LIFESTYLE

You cannot change the risk factors for colorectal cancer that involve your age, race, genetics, or family or personal medical history.

By being aware of these risk factors, however, you and your doctor can determine if you are at a higher risk for developing colorectal cancer, when to begin screening, and what the most appropriate method of screening is for you (see tables 4-1A,B for screening guidelines). Regardless of your risk level, the best way to prevent or improve your odds of survival from colorectal cancer is to get regular screenings (see chapters 3 and 4)—something I'll be harping on throughout this book.

Fortunately, there are risk factors you *can* control—those associated with your day-to-day habits and lifestyle. Improving your habits and lifestyle will reduce your risk of colorectal cancer while enhancing your overall health and sense of well-being.

Excess Weight

Emerging research shows that being very overweight increases your risk for colorectal cancer, although scientists are not sure why. One possible explanation is that excess weight is linked to the level of insulin-like growth factors in your body. These are hormones that may lead to the abnormal growth of cells in your colon and rectum.

Your risk of developing colorectal cancer is elevated, too, if excess fat is concentrated mostly around your waist. Studies suggest that abdominal fat alters your metabolism in a way that increases cell growth in the colon and rectum. If you're struggling with obesity, you can deal constructively with this risk factor by consulting your doctor and considering the diet and exercise guidelines in chapter 5.

Lack of Physical Activity

Numerous large-scale studies, including the famed Nurses' Health Study (which has followed and documented the nutrition and health habits of nearly ninety thousand nurses since 1976), have discovered that people who get little to no exercise are more susceptible to colon and rectal cancers than people who exercise daily.

Why is this?

For one thing, your bowel motility (the movement of material through your colon) is highly dependent on whether or not your entire body moves. The less active you are, the more sluggishly waste passes through your colon. This slowed movement may increase the time the lining of your colon is exposed to possible cancer-promoting agents. So if you rarely get exercise, you need to consult your doctor about starting a regimen that is appropriate for your fitness level.

Alcohol Consumption

You've no doubt heard the news that moderate drinking of certain types of alcohol, namely red wine, is beneficial to your heart and has been associated with other health benefits. This is because red wine contains a number of cell-protecting nutrients called antioxidants, which are also available from fruits and vegetables. However, there is no question that alcohol is harmful to your colon, and indeed to your entire gastrointestinal tract. Alcohol impairs bowel motility, harms the lining of the GI tract, and interferes with the absorption of certain nutrients (these effects go away when you stop drinking). Unfortunately, I've seen enough cirrhosis, pancreatic disease, and gastrointestinal hemorrhage in alcoholics to know that alcohol is not the life of the party.

Moderate alcohol usage (one drink per day) has been linked to an increased risk of colorectal cancer. This risk has been observed in people drinking mostly beer or hard liquor, more so than wine. Researchers aren't sure why drinking beer or hard liquor increases your risk for colorectal cancer, but they believe that abstaining from or limiting alcohol may protect levels of folic acid in the body. Folic acid is a B vitamin that may help prevent colon cells from turning cancerous.

Because too many unanswered questions remain, I believe that it's best not to recommend any amount of alcohol for medicinal purposes. There's no question in my mind of the damage excess or even moderate alcohol usage can inflict.

Long History of Smoking

People who have smoked for more than thirty-five years have an increased risk of dying from colorectal cancer—a 30 to 40 percent increase, according to the American Cancer Society. One study, conducted by researchers at the University of Utah, found that microsatellite instability, the genetic alteration I discussed previously, is strongly linked to smoking. MSI makes cells grow abnormally, developing into adenomatous polyps and eventually to cancer. The researchers discovered that colon cancer patients with MSI were those who smoked twenty or more cigarettes a day, began smoking at a young age, and had smoked for thirty-five years or more, compared to colon cancer patients without MSI. Thus, smoking appears to be a huge risk factor for MSI in tumors.

Diet

A growing catalog of studies suggests that diet plays a strong role in the risk of developing colorectal cancer. For example, people who eat a lot of plant-based foods each day, including fruits, vegetables, and whole grains, have a lower risk. Vegetables, in particular, are loaded with a wide range of protective agents, including folic acid, that guard against cancer.

Another dietary risk factor causing a lot of ruckus is red meat. Red meat has become a bad guy in the world of colorectal cancer—an indictment stemming from a number of large, credible studies suggesting that eating a lot of red meat is associated with an increased risk of the disease. Studies have shown that people who consume red meat five times a week have more than double the risk of colorectal cancer than people who eat these meats less than once a month.

Red meat is high in fat, and fat steps up the production of bile acid, which may be harmful to colon cells. What's more, red meat is high in iron—an important mineral, but one that in excess may generate damaging free radicals. For these reasons, an excess of red meat in the diet is believed to promote conditions favorable to colorectal cancer.

Marginal Deficiencies of Folic Acid

Much research suggests that the less folic acid in your diet, the higher your risk for colorectal cancer. An important B vitamin, folic acid is abundant in fruits, vegetables, and whole grains. If you're skimping on any of these foods, increasing your intake could help reduce your risk for colorectal cancer. Although I cover folic acid in detail in chapter 6, it is crucial to point out that you can obtain enough of this protective nutrient from foods and by taking a daily multivitamin containing 400 micrograms of folic acid. In fact, studies show that people who take a multivitamin with folic acid have a lower risk of colorectal cancer.

UNDERSTANDING YOUR RISK FACTORS

Looking over these risk factors, you can see which you can control or change and which you cannot control or change to help reduce your risk for developing colorectal cancer (see table 2-1). For example, you cannot change your age, genetics, or medical history, but you can strive to be healthier in the way that you eat, exercise, and live your life. In addition, by looking at all the risk factors for colorectal cancer you can see which factors place you at an *increased* risk for colorectal cancer, meaning that if you have these particular risk factors you may need to undergo screening for colorectal cancer at an earlier age or more frequently than those who do not have these particular risk factors. See table 2-2 to help you and your doctor determine whether you are at average or increased risk. If you want to jump ahead, tables 4-1A and 4-1B on pages 66 and 67 review currently recommended screening guidelines for colorectal cancer. Remember, in my book, regular screening is our most powerful weapon in treating—and preventing—colorectal cancer.

Table 2-1

Risk Factors for Colorectal Cancer

Factors You Cannot Control	Factors You Can Control
• Age.	• Diet.
• Hereditary or inherited syndromes.	• Weight.
• Family medical history.	• Physical activity.
• Personal medical history.	• Tobacco use.
	• Alcohol use.

Table 2-2

Risk Factors That Can Mean *Increased Risk* for Colorectal Cancer

Age

• Fifty years and older.

Hereditary or Inherited Syndromes

• Hereditary Nonpolyposis Colorectal Cancer (HNPCC).
• Familial Adenomatous Polyposis (FAP).

Family Medical History (First-, Second-, and Third-Degree Relatives*)

• Adenomatous polyps.[†]
• Colorectal cancer.[†]
• Other associated cancer, such as endometrial (uterine), ovarian, and stomach.[‡]

Personal Medical History

• Adenomatous polyps.
• Colorectal cancer.
• Inflammatory bowel disease (ulcerative colitis and Crohn's disease).
• Other associated cancer, such as endometrial (uterine), ovarian, and stomach.[‡]
• Breast cancer.[§]

*First-degree relatives include parents, siblings, and children. Second-degree relatives include grandparents, aunts, and uncles. Third-degree relatives include great-grandparents and cousins.

[†]This finding is more significant if the affected family member is a first-degree relative and was diagnosed before the age of fifty or if multiple first- or second-degree relatives have this finding.

[‡]These associated cancers are not labeled as increased risk in any of the formal guidelines for colorectal cancer screening. They may add risk, however, if they developed at a young age. In addition, these other cancers may raise a red flag for HNPCC.

[§]Emerging research suggests that there may be an increased risk for colorectal cancer in women who have had breast cancer.

Part II:

STOP COLORECTAL CANCER NOW: THE LIFESAVING POWER OF SCREENING AND PREVENTION

Chapter 3

The Colonoscopy: Your Most Powerful Weapon Against Colorectal Cancer

Your best chance of preventing colorectal cancer or detecting any colorectal cancer *early* is to undergo screening for the disease. When you undergo screening for colorectal cancer, this means that you have a test to detect polyps or cancer when you are feeling well—*before* any signs or symptoms of disease are present. The signs and symptoms of colorectal cancer (see sidebar, page 16) usually do not develop until the disease is more advanced, so getting tested when you are feeling well is essential to finding colorectal cancer early when it is most curable.

There are five different test options from which to choose when you undergo screening for colorectal cancer (see tables 4-1A,B). It is important that these different options are available, because not all health care facilities offer every test. My personal belief is that a colonoscopy is the most effective and comprehensive screening test currently available. This is because a colonoscopy allows your gastroenterologist or surgeon to view the inside of the entire colon and rectum, remove tissue for biopsy if needed, and remove polyps or early cancer if any is found—all during this one procedure.

Among the available screening tests for cancer, a colonoscopy is rather unique. It is the only screening procedure in which a doctor can not only detect the disease by finding a cancer, but also prevent it by removing a polyp, anywhere in the colon or rectum. Other medical screening tests such as a PSA for prostate cancer or a mammogram for breast cancer *can* find cancers in their earliest, most curable stages. Unlike a colonoscopy, however, these tests can neither prevent nor remove the cancer. They just detect it. If a polyp is found during a colonoscopy, it can be removed immediately, halting the possibility that it will turn into a cancer.

Sadly, many people never get screened for colorectal cancer and thus miss out on the single most powerful way to prevent this deadly disease. As a physician, it's frustrating to see this disease so frequently when it can be prevented with regular screening.

WHY PEOPLE DELAY OR PUT OFF SCREENING

One reason more people aren't being screened is that many doctors may neglect to recommend screening tests. Another is that there is a lot of confusion among doctors and their patients about which tests to have and when. But perhaps the greatest reason more people aren't being screened is that they are fearful or embarrassed about having the tests, especially since these tests involve the colon. In short, people just don't want to hear about having a tube placed in a very sensitive and embarrassing place—especially when they are feeling well. Consequently, doctors are diagnosing people at later stages of colorectal cancer, after it has spread beyond the colon when therapy is far less effective. That's a tragedy that just doesn't have to be.

Please don't let your anxiety or embarrassment rule your common sense. These fears are worth conquering if you realize that the chance of a cure is greater than 90 percent when colorectal cancer is detected and removed early.

Incidentally, age fifty is the magic number when it comes to screening and prevention. You should have your first screening and prevention test at age fifty, since the risk for colorectal cancer rises dramatically after that age. You may be at increased risk for colorectal cancer if you have a family history of polyps or cancer (not just colon cancer), so make sure you discuss this with your doctor. If you are at an increased risk, you should be screened earlier, more often, or both (see table 4-1B).

In this chapter, I'll discuss the colonoscopy in detail, and in the next chapter I'll cover other screening options, including the fecal occult blood test (FOBT), flexible sigmoidoscopy, double contrast barium enema, and digital rectal exam. Which one is right for you? In the words of Dr. Sidney Winawer, the primary investigator of the prestigious National Polyp Study: "The right screening test for you is *the one that gets done!*"

That said, let's start by talking about the amazing procedure known as a colonoscopy.

THE COLONOSCOPY

What It Is

A colonoscopy is a medical procedure that involves advancing a special instrument called a colonoscope through the rectum and the entire length of your colon while you are sedated. The purpose of a screening colonoscopy is to find polyps and cancer and to remove them whenever possible.

The removal of a polyp during a colonoscopy is medically termed a polypectomy. (A polypectomy can also be performed during a flexible sigmoidoscopy, which is discussed in the next chapter, or during surgery, although this type of operation is rare.)

Who Performs This Test

There are two types of medical doctors you can see for this procedure: gastroenterologists and surgeons. Physicians who perform colonoscopies should be board-certified in their specialty. Equally important, they should be well trained and experienced in performing colonoscopies. The initial stage of finding such a doctor may involve a referral from your own family doctor, or you can ask friends, family, or a local medical center for names of doctors who have the experience and training you are looking for. To my knowledge the only organization that requires proof of training in endoscopic procedures such as colonoscopies is the American Society for Gastrointestinal Endoscopy (ASGE), which has a Web site at www.asge.org. If you need to find a doctor to do a colonoscopy and can't get an appropriate recommendation, this is a good place to start.

Colonoscopies are performed in hospitals, clinics, outpatient surgery centers, endoscopy facilities, and private doctors' offices. If you are elderly or medically ill, I recommend having the procedure in a hospital because support services are available, in the unlikely event of an emergency. If you are otherwise healthy and undergoing screening, any approved facility is fine.

Most often, the physician performing your colonoscopy or a trained nurse will administer the sedation. In certain situations, there will be a separate anesthesiologist to perform a deeper sedation. Assisting your doctor with the procedure will be a nurse and/ or technician.

Consultation Before the Test

Prior to having your colonoscopy, you should speak or meet with the examining physician or assistant for a consultation. At that time, a detailed medical history will be taken to learn whether you have any allergies to medications or anesthesia; bleeding problems; or other diseases or conditions that may affect the procedure.

Certain medications may need to be changed or stopped before a colonoscopy. The most worrisome types of medications are those that interfere with blood clotting because they may increase the risk of bleeding if a polyp is removed or a biopsy performed. The list of "blood thinners" is long and includes Coumadin (warfarin), Lovenox (enoxparin), Plavix (clopidogrel), aspirin, and all non-steroidal anti-inflammatory drugs (NSAIDs). NSAIDs include over-the-counter and prescription medications such as Motrin and Advil (ibuprofen) and Aleve (naproxyn). If you are on any of these medications or others, please discuss with your doctor what needs to be done before the colonoscopy. Often, your doctor will want you to stop the medication five to seven days before the procedure. Talk to your doctor well before that time frame so you know exactly what needs to be changed with your medication.

During this consultation, your doctor will also discuss with you the risks and benefits of the procedure and explain the pre-procedure preparation. He or she should also explain that a colonoscopy does not hurt because you are sedated; you really should not feel any discomfort at all. The overall purpose of this consultation is for you to understand the procedure. Any caring doctor should be able to reassure you and make you feel comfortable about having a colonoscopy.

The Informed Consent

You'll be asked to sign a consent form during your consultation or immediately before the procedure. This is not a legal document! The consent form only assures that a conversation took place about procedure risks and benefits. Even so, many patients respond to this form by thinking, *I am signing my life away*, but nothing could be further from the truth. There are some known risks to the procedure that I will discuss, but the lifesaving benefits certainly outweigh any of the theoretical risks. You are not signing your life away but doing just the opposite—protecting it!

The Colonoscopy Bowel Preparation

Your doctor will give you specific instructions on how to prepare for your colonoscopy during the initial consultation. The preparation, or prep, for a colonoscopy is absolutely crucial and, without a doubt, the worst part of the whole colonoscopy procedure. Its purpose is to completely clean your colon of any fecal material so that your doctor has a crystal-clear view of its internal lining. In fact, once the prep is complete, your colon will look almost as clean as the lining of your mouth. People think of a colonoscopy as a dirty and disgusting procedure. As you will learn, however, this is just not the case. If you are awake enough to watch the procedure or look at photographs afterward, you will see firsthand how clean and interesting your colon appears.

The prep involves a special diet and the use of oral laxatives beginning the day before your colonoscopy. There is no pain or cramping involved with the prep, just a lot of trips to the bathroom. Some people complain about feeling nauseated after taking the laxatives. Only infrequently does the nausea lead to vomiting. Even so, the laxatives are usually at work by the time the vomiting occurs. So don't worry if you didn't keep the laxatives down—you will still see their effects.

Most people can go about their normal activities the day before the procedure while on the liquid diet. The oral laxatives are usually not started until the late afternoon or the early evening prior to the colonoscopy. Once the laxative is taken, response time is varied. Most people begin to get diarrhea one to two hours after the first dose. However, there are those few individuals who do not start seeing an effect until the laxative has been completely finished. Trust me on this one—I have never seen an individual who did not develop diarrhea after the bowel prep . . . it just takes some people longer than others.

THE CLEAR LIQUID DIET

The most widely used diet for colon preparation is a clear liquid diet, which you'll follow the day before you have your colonoscopy. On this diet, you eat and drink clear liquids only. These include:

- Chicken or beef broth (not bouillon because it can leave residue in your colon).
- Yellow Jell-O (not red Jell-O as this may look like blood in the colon).
- Clear fruit juice, such as white grape juice, white cranberry juice, or apple juice.
- Water.
- Flavored waters.
- Coffee or tea, black or with sugar (although I personally don't think a drop of milk really makes a difference).

So that you don't feel deprived or hungry during the day of your prep, it is a good idea to fix yourself a big bowl of Jell-O, along with a large bowl of broth and a tall glass of clear fruit juice, for breakfast, lunch, and dinner. Chicken broth is a particularly good choice

does. You drink approximately a gallon of PEG-containing fluid in order to flush out your digestive system.

At least fifteen hours prior to your colonoscopy, you start drinking this laxative eight ounces at a time, every fifteen minutes, until you finish the entire container. It tastes unpleasant due to its active ingredient, polyethylene glycol, which chemically is not much different than radiator fluid. One trick here is to keep it ice cold so that your taste buds are not as sensitive to the flavor. If possible, drink at least two more eight-ounce glasses of water the night before having the procedure. As with the sodium phosphate prep, a clear liquid diet must be followed starting the day before your colonoscopy.

The Pill Laxative Prep

Your doctor may not have told you about the pill prep because it's fairly new on the scene, but patients are often asking about it. Basically, this is the pill form of the active ingredient (sodium phosphate) in Fleet Phospho-Soda and is known commercially as Visicol. Visicol is available by prescription only. Unfortunately, it takes a lot of pills to match the concentration of liquid sodium phosphate. The prep procedure includes taking:

- Four pills taken every fifteen minutes a total of five times the night before your colonoscopy (for a total of twenty pills throughout the evening).
- Four pills, taken fifteen minutes apart, for a total of eight pills in the morning.
- Each set of four pills is taken with eight ounces of clear liquid such as water, juice, ginger ale, or sports drink (not red).

This regimen will evacuate your colon in time for your test. While taking this laxative, you must follow the clear liquid diet previously discussed.

Although the major advantage of the pill prep is that you do not need to taste the Phospho-Soda, there is a slight downside to this prep from a doctor's standpoint. A small amount of pill residue known as microcrystalline cellulose (MCC) may remain in your colon, particularly in the cecum and right side of the colon. Your doctor will need to clear the view, and this can prolong the procedure.

As with the Phospho-Soda, you should not take Visicol if you are elderly or have kidney conditions, heart trouble, or a history of dehydration.

OTHER PREPS

Alternative bowel-cleansing preparations are being developed and introduced all the time, in the hope that easier, less objectionable preps will encourage more people to have colonoscopies. One of the newer preps is the LoSo Prep System. It consists of the following laxatives: magnesium citrate, a liquid oral laxative with a citrus flavor; four bisacodyl tablets, both taken the day before your colonoscopy; and one bisacodyl suppository, used on the morning of the procedure.

Another alternative is the MiraLax prep. MiraLax is a lower dose of PEG-containing powder that dissolves in water. Like other PEG-containing laxatives, MiraLax is not absorbed from the intestinal tract, but stays within the gut to hold water inside the intestine, thereby increasing the volume and frequency of bowel movements. When MiraLax is used as a colonoscopy prep, you usually mix it with sixty-four ounces of a sports drink and take it in conjunction with other laxatives.

Alternative to the Clear Liquid Diet: The Low-Residue Diet

Designed to replace the clear liquid diet is something relatively new: the low-residue diet, marketed as the NutraPrep Meal Kit. You follow this diet, along with one of the prep choices previously described.

The low-residue diet contains a full day's worth of nutritional shakes, soups, energy bars, and chips, all specially prepared to provide essential nutrition, plus significantly reduce the amount of residue remaining in your colon after digestion. While following this one-day diet, you eat specific foods at certain times during the day.

The low-residue diet has significant advantages because it does not cause the weakness, hunger, and irritability often associated with the clear liquid diet. Time, experience, and research will tell if this diet is as good as the standard clear liquids currently recommended by most physicians.

If you feel that you cannot tolerate clear liquids for a day, ask your doctor about this dietary preparation, and whether it can be prescribed for you. Because it is so new, your doctor may not be familiar with it.

What Your Doctor May Not Have Told You: Other Strategies for Surviving Your Colonoscopy Prep

▪ *Have some flushable moist wipes on hand:* Normal toilet paper can be very abrasive and, believe me, you are going to need quite a bit of it. Buy moist flushable wipes (usually located in the hemorrhoid ointment section of your grocery of drugstore) or flushable baby wipes to use in place of toilet paper.

▪ *Use hemorrhoid ointment:* Don't wait for your bottom to become sore. One easy early intervention is to use a hemorrhoid ointment after each bowel movement. I recommend Nupercainal because it has a local anesthetic in a petroleum jelly base.

▪ *Get a good book or magazine to read while on the toilet:* You may as well enjoy your time in the bathroom.

Sedation and Your Colonoscopy

Most colonoscopies are performed under a type of mild anesthesia known as conscious sedation. This means that you are in a twilight state where you feel comfortable, relaxed, and euphoric. In this condition, you just want to close your eyes and sleep.

Conscious sedation also interferes with the function of your memory and creates an amnesia-like state. In fact, it can be so powerful that some patients may insist that the colonoscopy never took place, when in fact it had already been completed. All in all, sedation really is quite a relaxing and enjoyable experience for many patients.

Typically, this type of sedation consists of intravenous Demerol (meperidine), a narcotic painkiller similar to morphine, and Versed (midazolam), a sedative similar to Valium (diazepam). A shorter-acting narcotic called fentanyl may be substituted for Demerol in certain cases.

A deeper form of sedation, which I call unconscious sedation, puts you completely "out." Unconscious sedation is different from general anesthesia because you continue breathing on your own, without the need for any mechanical assistance such as a respirator. The drug used for this sedation is propofol (Diprivan), a new kid on the block for procedures requiring deep sedation. This drug is a very powerful sedative-hypnotic. Because of the potency of this drug, it can be administered only by specially trained nurses, doctors, and anesthesiologists. It may not even be available from your doctor. I selectively use propofol on patients who have had difficulty with sedation in the past, require long or complicated procedures, are taking pain medications or sedatives, or drink alcohol regularly.

Under the influence of propofol, you remember nothing about the procedure, and experience no time lapse between going to sleep and waking up. As one patient told his doctor: "It does feel weird. You go to sleep in one room and then you wake up in a totally different room. Just like college." All kidding aside, a huge advantage of propofol—and the reason why more and more doctors are using it—is that it creates a deep level of sedation and does not produce as much postoperative grogginess that is so often associated with other sedative agents.

Whatever sedation is used, you should not experience any discomfort or pain during your colonoscopy. Every patient of mine says the exact same thing when we finish: "That's it? We're done? That was the big deal?" Most people who have had colonoscopies will say that the procedure is a piece of cake. It is the prep that is annoying.

The Procedure

The instrument used in a colonoscopy is called a colonoscope, which consists of a long flexible tube that is the thickness of a finger. It contains a light; a video camera; an air insufflation device to release air into the colon; a lens irrigator; and a hollow channel to suction liquid and pass therapeutic instruments such as biopsy forceps and polyp removal devices. The fact that these slender scopes can hold all this technology is really quite amazing.

During the colonoscopy, this instrument is gently placed into the rectum, advanced through the colon, and then slowly withdrawn. During that time, your doctor is looking for polyps, cancers, and other abnormalities. If a polyp is found, it is removed right then and there.

The best view of the colon occurs while the instrument is being withdrawn. That is because the scope is moving in the same direction that fecal matter moves, and thus the colon is accustomed to this direction. By contrast, when the scope is advanced from the rectum to the cecum—the origin of the colon—it is really traveling down a one-way street, the wrong way. Consequently, the colon often contracts against the scope, attempting to push this foreign device out. Upon withdrawal, however, the colon is more relaxed, and the lining is easily evaluated.

Your doctor looks at the lining of your colon on a television monitor. The image comes from the tip of the colonoscope. Many patients may be awake enough, especially during the withdrawal, to watch the procedure on the same monitor that the doctor uses.

Although your first impression may be *Ugh,* most patients find the experience simply fascinating. Remember, everything is clean inside the colon after the prep. As comedian Robin Williams once put it, "It is like watching your own private Discovery Channel."

Your doctor controls the colonoscope's progress through your colon with two dials. One dial moves the tip up and down, while the other moves it left and right. Pictures are taken along the way, and you can get your own souvenir copies later, if you wish (I usually autograph my patients' photos).

During the procedure, air may be pumped through the colonoscope into your colon to inflate the colon for a better view. The colonoscope is also capable of suctioning out any residual secretions and stool that may obstruct the view. Patients are often concerned that they are not "cleaned out enough." As long as any residue is liquid, it can be suctioned out.

If polyps or suspicious growths are observed along the way, they can be removed either with a device called a snare, or with a biopsy forceps. The snare is a small lasso-like device that is tightened like a noose around the base of a polyp. Once the snare is tight, electric current is applied that converts this metal loop into a cutting device that burns (cauterizes) tissue through the base of the polyp until it falls off. Smaller polyps may be removed in this manner without current or with a device known as a hot biopsy forceps. This device grabs the polyp with tiny pincers; when electric current is applied, the polyp is burned off. The tiniest polyps are usually removed through simple biopsy without electricity. All tissue removed is sent to a pathology lab for evaluation.

Risks

Most invasive medical procedures entail a degree of risk, and a colonoscopy is no exception. Thus, it is important to recognize the potential risks of this procedure. For perspective, however, every individual has about a 6 percent lifetime risk of developing colorectal cancer. This incidence is clearly outweighed by the potential benefit of preventing a deadly disease through a colonoscopy. I honestly believe that crossing York Avenue in New York City to get to my endoscopy suite is probably a riskier event than having a colonoscopy.

PERFORATION

Colonoscopies carry a higher risk of bowel perforation than do other screening methods. However, these are very rare—one in thousands. In fact, I believe that the risk of this complication in otherwise healthy patients undergoing screening colonoscopies is even less than what is currently thought.

These rare perforations can occur if the colonoscope loops as it navigates its way around the hairpinlike turn in the sigmoid portion of the colon. Keeping the colonoscope as straight as possible during the procedure reduces this problem, however.

Another cause of perforation is the infused air used during the procedure. In someone who has diverticulosis—the presence of small bulges called diverticula in the colon—the air can perforate a diverticulum. But again, this complication is exceedingly rare. If a perforation does occur, it may heal on its own with appropriate treatment, or surgery may be required. Fortunately, since the bowel is already prepped, surgery can often be done in a minimally invasive manner utilizing a rather new procedure called laparoscopy (see chapter 9 for a full description of this). But, as I tell my patients, the chances of having a bowel perforation are extremely low—so know about it, but certainly don't worry about it.

BLEEDING

If a polyp is removed, there may be bleeding at the removal site, but this occurs very infrequently. Bleeding, however, can be easily controlled and cauterized directly at the site.

After the polyp is removed, a small risk of bleeding can remain for up to two weeks. This may occur if the healing site sloughs its surface, much like a cut having its scab knocked off. The possibility of bleeding is one reason why doctors often ask their patients to avoid aspirin and anti-inflammatory drugs before the procedure, since these drugs may interfere with normal blood clotting. Even if this happens, the bleeding often stops on its own. In the worst of cases, another colonoscopy procedure can be performed to cauterize the site. So again, don't spend too much time worrying about this.

SEDATION RISKS

Although uncommon, an adverse reaction to the sedation could occur. Sedation typically lowers the amount of oxygen in the blood because the breathing becomes more relaxed. Rarely, the respiration becomes so relaxed that breathing support has to be given with a device called an ambu bag. Many endoscopy suites now use supplemental oxygen as a nasal cannula (small device placed under the nose) before the sedation is even given to ensure adequate oxygen levels. In order to monitor the exact blood oxygen amount, a small device is put on the finger or ear that actually measures blood oxygen saturation by analyzing how red the blood is (the technology is amazing!). Blood low in oxygen, such as that in your veins, is blue; blood rich in oxygen, such as the blood in your arteries, is red.

UNDETECTED POLYPS AND CANCER

Nothing in medicine is 100 percent. There is a slight risk (about 6 percent) that some polyps or small cancers won't be detected during a colonoscopy—for three main reasons.

First, the anatomy of the colon may not permit the scope to see into every "nook and cranny"—even in the most skilled of hands. Thus, something small may go undetected.

Second, on rare occasions, the colonoscope may not physically reach the origin of the colon. This is known as an incomplete colonoscopy and can be due to a very long looping colon that just will not allow safe passage of the colonoscope to its far reaches. In fact, you may hear your doctor use the words *redundant* or *tortuous* when describing someone's colon. This simply means that the colon is long, floppy, and curving.

Third, a poor prep or difficulty with sedation may interfere with the doctor's ability to complete the procedure.

These situations, however, occur infrequently and are not a cause for alarm.

After the Test

Following your colonoscopy, you will be kept under observation until the sedation wears off, and someone will have to pick you up and drive you home. You may feel some mild cramping due to the air that was placed in your colon at the time of the procedure. Fortunately, the body has a very good and natural way of expelling this gas, so don't be bashful about letting it do its thing. This may be the only time it is socially acceptable to pass gas, so enjoy it!

Because sedation temporarily interferes with memory, there have been times when I've had full conversations with patients only to find out later that they were upset that I never "spoke to them after the procedure." So, I have two suggestions. First, make sure somebody is with you when the doctor discusses the findings of your colonoscopy. Second, don't get upset with your doctor if you believe that he or she never talked with you after the procedure—perhaps you just don't remember.

After the procedure, you need to drink lots of fluids to replace those lost by the laxatives you took during your prep. Generally, you can resume a normal diet, but it is best to eat a softer diet than usual for at least one day after the procedure. You should rest after your colonoscopy and resume your normal activities and exercise a day later.

Alert: If you run a fever, have chills, experience severe abdominal cramps, have pronounced rectal bleeding, or experience a combination of these, call your doctor immediately. These symptoms may indicate a perforation or other serious complication.

What Your Results Mean

The doctor who performed your colonoscopy will often talk to you afterward about what was found and whether a polyp was removed. Usually, a doctor will know if a polyp or a growth may be serious. A final answer cannot be given, however, until the pathologic evaluation of the tissue is performed. That is why a doctor will ask that you call the office to get the final results—it does *not* mean that your doctor suspects something abnormal. If a doctor tells you the polyp looks benign (not cancerous), he or she is probably right.

If a polyp or other tissue was removed during the procedure, it will be sent to a pathology lab for examination. A normal, or negative result, means that nothing suspicious or abnormal was found.

A positive result indicates that polyps, tumors, or other suspicious-looking growths were detected in the lining of your colon or rectum. If cancerous cells are found in the tissue sample, then a diagnosis of colon or rectal cancer is made. You'll learn more about pathology, biopsies, and results in chapter 7.

Other abnormal findings that might be discussed include hemorrhoids, inflammation, diverticulosis, inflammatory bowel disease, and vascular abnormalities. These are viewed directly during the colonoscopy.

Usually, you'll be asked to call in about a week to find out your biopsy or polyp results. Most doctors will discuss the results over the phone and tell you when you need a follow-up colonoscopy (usually between three to ten years). However, if there is any concern about the findings or pathology results, it is best to have this discussion in person. Often this type of more serious news is expected based on the findings seen at the colonoscopy. In my practice, if something suspicious is found during the procedure, I usually schedule a follow-up visit in my office so that I can discuss any potential bad news in person. Some doctors discuss *all* results in person, so don't get frightened if you are told to come back to the office after the procedure.

Very important: Suppose your colonoscopy reveals an adenomatous (potentially precancerous) polyp. What your doctor may not tell you—but should—is this: "Given the results of your colonoscopy, if you have any brothers, sisters, or children, they all need to discuss colorectal cancer screening with their doctors, even if they are younger than age fifty." This is a vital part of the doctor–patient conversation *that often gets omitted.* You need to have this discussion with your doctor so that you can help protect your family from colorectal cancer. What I tell my patients is that I view a polyp as a family problem. If you have one, then so can others in your family. So please make sure your family is informed about your polyp so that they can get the appropriate screening for themselves.

Remember: You owe it to yourself and your loved ones to get screened. Don't delay; make your appointment today. *A colonoscopy is the only screening procedure that detects polyps and tumors through the entire length of your colon. It is truly a lifesaving procedure.* Trust me on this: I have personally seen this procedure save many lives.

Although I believe a colonoscopy is the best method of screening and prevention, there are other screening technologies in use. Let's take a closer look at those.

Chapter 4

Other Screening Techniques

Other valuable screening tests for colorectal cancer are available, some of which should be a part of your annual physical. Though not as accurate as a colonoscopy, the procedures discussed below have their place in colorectal cancer detection and are often used in conjunction with a colonoscopy.

FECAL OCCULT BLOOD TEST (FOBT)

What It Is

The presence of microscopic blood in your stool is one of many indicators of colon or rectal cancer (but hardly the most definitive). Both cancers and polyps can cause a small amount of bleeding, which can turn up in your stool. Usually, this blood cannot be seen in the stool and is termed occult blood. This easy, inexpensive, and painless test looks for such blood and should be performed routinely as part of your annual physical examination. There is really no excuse not to do this one. In fact, this is the exact test that first discovered former president Ronald Reagan's colon cancer. Research shows that an annual FOBT can reduce deaths from colorectal cancer by 33 percent. FOBT is currently the only test that has been studied long enough to demonstrate a decrease in colorectal death rates.

Why does it work so well?

I believe it works because of early cancer detection and the removal of polyps by colonoscopy. Any positive result of the FOBT requires a colonoscopy to look for the source of blood. Most FOBT positive results do not turn up any cancer, but if a polyp is found at the time of colonoscopy, it is removed. So a percentage of people who have a FOBT test performed will require colonoscopy.

Who Performs This Test

This is a test that you can get from your doctor, bring home, and perform yourself by collecting several stool samples from three consecutive bowel movements and smearing them on special cards. Make sure that you take all three stool samples, because polyps and cancers tend to bleed intermittently.

There are several take-home tests available on the market that you can purchase at pharmacies, but I advise that you check with your doctor to find out which ones are clinically accurate, or if you should even use such a test. Cancer isn't a disease you should try to diagnose yourself. Keep in mind that these over-the-counter tests are not as reliable at detecting early-stage colorectal cancer or precancerous polyps as the screening tests your doctor can do. And they are certainly not a replacement for your doctor's diagnosis.

Before the Test

During the days when you perform this test, you must avoid red meat, citrus fruit, radishes, vitamin C supplements, aspirin, iron, and other substances known to sway the results. Read the test instructions carefully, noting foods, medications, and supplements that you should avoid, because your doctor may not fully inform you about these.

How FOBT Works

The card is impregnated with a substance called guaiac, a tree bark extract. When hydrogen peroxide is added to the card, a reaction occurs. If hidden blood is present in detectable amounts, the card will turn blue within about thirty seconds. With the take-home FOBT test, you simply toss the test tissues into the toilet bowl and wait to see if they turn blue.

Risks

This test is risk-free. The major drawback is that it is easy to make mistakes when performing the test at home. Still, even if you unknowingly mess up the test and it turns out positive, your doctor will insist that you undergo a colonoscopy, especially if you're age fifty or over. That's a good thing, really, since a colonoscopy is the most accurate screening test available. One other risk with the FOBT is that polyps and even cancers may still exist in the setting of a negative FOBT. That is why this test must be done every year and is often combined with other tests.

After the Test

When you're finished with the test, take the sample card back to your doctor, or mail it to a laboratory to be analyzed for blood. If you used a home test purchased at the pharmacy and you think it indicated blood in your stool, talk to your doctor about having a more definitive procedure.

What Your Results Mean

If the card turns blue (a positive result), you will need a colonoscopy to look for polyps or cancer in your colon and rectum. FOBT is known to produce many positive results that are not caused by polyps or cancer (false positives). Blood in the stool may be caused by other conditions, such as hemorrhoids or inflammation. Stomach ulcers can also cause blood in your stool, so you may have to be examined for this condition as well with an upper endoscopy (a procedure that views the upper portion of your gastrointestinal tract, including your stomach). An upper endoscopy can be performed at the same time as a colonoscopy. Finally, false positives may be caused by food that was eaten, such as red meat. If your FOBT is negative, repeat it a year later, unless you are scheduled to have a colonoscopy.

FLEXIBLE SIGMOIDOSCOPY

What It Is

The flexible sigmoidoscopy is a screening procedure used to find colorectal cancer and polyps in the rectum and lower part of the colon; to pinpoint the cause of rectal bleeding, or diarrhea; or to diagnose certain types of inflammatory bowel disease. It investigates only the rectum and sigmoid colon—the portion of the colon located between the descending colon (in the left side of the abdomen) and the rectum. Any polyps detected can be removed during the procedure.

I want to be upfront and honest with you about this procedure: Where colorectal cancer detection is concerned, this exam has fallen out of favor because it does not examine the entire colon and therefore can miss polyps and tumors. In my opinion, it's like doing a mammogram on one breast. You never get the full picture. So if your doctor recommends this test and can't give a good reason why, you may want to request a colonoscopy instead.

Who Performs This Test

Flexible sigmoidoscopies are usually performed by primary care physicians or gastroenterologists and are conducted in a doctor's office or at a health clinic, outpatient surgery center, or hospital.

Before the Test

The preparation for a flexible sigmoidoscopy helps clean the lower portion of the colon so that your doctor can better see the lining. Several different bowel preparations are used for this test, so follow your doctor's instructions carefully. Usually, you'll have one or two enemas a few hours before the test to clean out the lower portion of your colon.

How It Works

You are usually not sedated for this procedure, so it can be a bit uncomfortable. Your doctor will insert a flexible fiber-optic tube into your rectum to examine the lower portion of your colon. Basically the flexible sigmoidoscope is a short colonoscope with the same type of light, camera, air, and biopsy channel. This instrument comes in two lengths, thirty-five and sixty centimeters (about fourteen and twenty-four inches, respectively); the longer model is better at detecting disease because it sees more of the lower colon. While the tube is being inserted, air is pumped into your bowel in order to distend the colon so that the tube can be positioned properly. This will produce some cramping and the urge to expel gas (remember, you are not sedated). Breathing deeply will ease these feelings.

If you wish, you can watch the images on a screen as the procedure is performed. The exam takes roughly ten to fifteen minutes.

Risks

There is a slight risk of perforation, although this is exceedingly rare. If a polyp is removed, there may also be a slight risk of bleeding, similar to the risk I described in the previous chapter.

After the Test

No special aftercare is required. If you have any unusual bleeding or pain, a call to your doctor is imperative.

What Your Results Mean

If your doctor detects any polyps or other suspicious growths, you'll need to be scheduled for a full colonoscopy. Typically, when growths are found in the portion of the colon screened by a flexible sigmoidoscopy, there's a good chance that there are polyps or growths in other parts of the colon as well.

DOUBLE CONTRAST BARIUM ENEMA

What It Is

This is one of the oldest tests used to evaluate the colon. The double contrast barium enema has been used to investigate abdominal pain, unusual bowel habits, diarrhea, chronic constipation, blood or mucus in the stool, and diseases of the colon and rectum, including cancer.

With this test, barium is given via an enema, and X rays are taken of the inside of your colon to look for polyps, cancer, and disease. Like the flexible sigmoidoscopy, this test has fallen out of favor for colorectal cancer detection because it is uncomfortable and fails to detect small polyps. And if anything is seen—guess what?—you still need a colonoscopy, because no growths can be removed or biopsied during this test. In a recently published article in the *New England Journal of Medicine,* the barium enema was found to be inferior to the colonoscopy for detecting polyps and growths.

Who Performs This Test

A barium enema is performed by radiologists, usually in the radiology department of a hospital or clinic. The art of the barium enema is being lost, however, because radiologists are performing fewer of these tests and are therefore less skilled in detecting polyps. So ask your doctor which radiologists in your area are the most experienced at performing this procedure.

Before the Test

The day before you have the test, you'll stop eating solid food and drink only clear liquids instead. You'll also take a laxative to clear out your intestinal tract. This laxative is not quite as powerful or as intense as the one given for a colonoscopy.

Just before the test, you'll be given a cleansing enema. During the actual test, you'll be given another enema using a tube that contains barium, a contrast agent through which X rays cannot pass. This material coats and fills in the hollows of your lower digestive tract and, with the addition of air, reveal a clear silhouette of the colon's shape and condition. This image lets the radiologist view large polyps or cancers.

How It Works

You will be asked to lie down on a special table, and the radiologist will press gently on your abdomen to direct the barium to your colon. Air will be forced through the enema tube into your colon during the X ray to expand it and improve the image seen on the X rays. The radiologist will move you back and forth on the table in different positions in order to obtain multiple views of your colon and abdomen. During the test, you will feel crampy, with the urge to defecate.

Risks

This test is virtually risk-free, although a barium enema can aggravate ulcerative colitis or irritate the lining of your colon. Bowel perforations due to the air have been reported, although this is exceedingly rare.

After the Test

After the X rays are taken, you'll be allowed to go to the bathroom to expel the barium. It is important that you drink plenty of liquids during the day to help expel any residual barium. Your stools may be white or pinkish for a few days after the procedure, or until the barium has completely exited your system.

What Your Results Mean

A barium enema can reveal a number of abnormalities, including large polyps, tumors, diverticulosis, ulcerative colitis, narrowing of the colon, and other diseases of the colon. If polyps or tumors are found, you'll have to undergo a colonoscopy or have surgery.

DIGITAL RECTAL EXAM

What It Is

Prior to the development of FOBT and other sophisticated screening tests, this exam was the only screening test available for detecting rectal cancer during routine physical examinations. Because this test is far less accurate than other screening procedures, though, it is no longer recommended for routine screening by itself, but used in conjunction with the FOBT.

Who Performs This Test

This test is performed by your primary care physician, or by a gastroenterologist or surgeon just before a colonoscopy to feel for growths.

Before the Test

No special preparation is necessary.

How It Works

Your doctor inserts a gloved finger into your rectum to feel for abnormal growths. This exam is also used as part of routine screening for prostate cancer.

Risks

None.

After the Test

No special aftercare is required.

What Your Results Mean

If any abnormality is found, your doctor will follow up with a flexible sigmoidoscopy or colonoscopy. If something is felt very close to the anus, a special instrument may be required to evaluate the area.

NEW TESTS ON THE HORIZON

Early detection will always be the best way to increase your chance of preventing or surviving colorectal cancer. As I've emphasized, far too many people skip screening procedures such as colonoscopies, because they are invasive and involve an uncomfortable bowel preparation. New screening procedures may well change all that.

Virtual Colonoscopy

This test clearly wins the Coolest Name Award. It sounds so high-tech and technical that it *must* be the best test, right? Well, the verdict is not yet in, but this exam is certainly generating a lot of excitement.

In this procedure, a device is inserted only at the opening of the rectum, where a large balloon is inflated to fill the viewing area with air so that the colon and rectum can be viewed with a computerized tomography (CT) scanner. Special computer software transforms the CT scan into a three-dimensional view of the colon and rectum. Just as in a video game, the radiologist can "travel" through the virtual colon using a joystick looking for polyps and cancer. No tube is threaded through your colon, making the virtual colonoscopy much less invasive, with little risk of bowel injury or bleeding. Some researchers have likened the virtual procedure to a mammogram of the colon.

The problem is that, in order to get the best look at the colon, you must still follow the identical bowel prep you used for a conventional colonoscopy. In addition, if a polyp or growth is found, you then must have a colonoscopy and take the prep again. So why not just have the colonoscopy—which can be both diagnostic *and* therapeutic—in the first place?

A recent study published in the *New England Journal of Medicine* showed that virtual colonoscopy is as accurate as regular colonoscopy for detecting polyps and cancer. However, it is not yet known if these results are reproducible in private radiology centers. This test raises an important question: Do all polyps discovered in a virtual colonoscopy need to be removed as they are with regular colonoscopy? If so, greater than 30 percent of all virtual colonoscopies will require a regular colonoscopy to remove polyps.

There is another important issue—insurance. At the time of this writing, virtual colonoscopy is not recognized as a well-studied and approved means of colon cancer screening and consequently is not covered by any insurance. This means that you must pay for this test out of pocket. The test costs about $500 to $1,000.

Even so, I do believe virtual colonoscopy has an important role now. Remember, for technical and safety reasons, not every colonoscopy can be completed. Sometimes a large growth might hinder the passage of the colonoscope through the colon, or the patient may have a hard-to-scope looping colon, as I explained earlier. In such cases, a doctor could immediately perform a virtual colonoscopy, since the patient is already prepped, and thus view the part of the colon that is otherwise not viewable.

Fecal DNA Testing

These new tests work by analyzing the DNA that is shed in stool, thereby identifying various genetic mutations that can lead to the development of colorectal cancer. Using the most modern genetic techniques currently available, scientists have developed a means of isolating—from the billions of DNA fragments found in stool—

only those specific DNA strands that are released by polyps and cancer. Imagine being able to find a single individual at a football game by analyzing the air over the stadium and detecting a molecule of air that was exhaled by that person. This is about how precise the test is from the technical standpoint.

But as amazing as it is, stool genetic testing can detect only about 65 percent of large polyps and cancers. So there is a substantial miss rate, and for this reason I still recommend colonoscopy.

The major advantage of this test over other stool tests is that a positive result almost always means that there is a large polyp or cancer. So if the test is positive, then you must undergo a colonoscopy to find out why. Unlike FOBT—which results in many false positive tests—stool genetic testing has very few false positives.

An appropriate role for this test right now may be in patients who just will not get a colonoscopy no matter what. At least this test will pick up half or more of significant polyps and cancer. In the future, this test may also be appropriate for people younger than fifty. Currently, there are no recommendations for screening this age group because the costs and risks do not outweigh the benefits. Still, about thirteen thousand people below the age of fifty are diagnosed with colon cancer each year. Perhaps this test, with its low false positive rate, can fill that gap. Further investigation needs to be done to see if this strategy makes sense.

Because of the laborious process to isolate DNA, and the patents on many of the genes being evaluated, the test (known as PreGen-Plus) costs about $500 to $750. Like the virtual colonoscopy, it is not yet covered by any insurance. What's more, it needs to be further studied and compared to other accepted screening options.

Even so, I believe fecal DNA testing represents one of the most exciting areas of colorectal cancer screening at present. A number of new DNA tests are being developed and tested, and I look forward to evaluating them in clinical trials.

The future of cancer testing lies in genetic evaluation. One day this approach may be so good that it could even be an alternative to the colonoscopy. That day is still years away, however, so don't wait.

Fecal Immunohistochemical Test (FIT)

Recently introduced, FIT is a newer, more accurate type of fecal stool test than the standard guaiac fecal occult blood test. In early testing, FIT was found to be significantly better at detecting cancers.

With FIT, you swish an instrument that looks like a watercolor paintbrush in the toilet water after a bowel movement on two separate occasions. This technique is easier than what is required for the FOBT, and it seems to be better accepted by patients. Researchers hope that the FIT will help increase the number of patients who get screened for colorectal cancer, and that the test will be better at picking up patients with microscopic blood in the stool. More research is required to validate this technique as a screening option.

Pill Endoscopy

Can you imagine swallowing a pill the size of a multivitamin that takes fifty thousand pictures of your intestine and sends those images wirelessly to a small hard drive attached to your waist? Capsule endoscopy actually exists and is currently being used to evaluate disorders of the small intestine. Every patient who hears about this new test calls my office and asks if they can do this test instead of the colonoscopy.

Unfortunately, the answer is no, and there are two reasons why. First, the battery in the capsule does not last long enough to reach the large intestine. Second, the colon is filled with stool and cannot be distended with air, so the capsule becomes coated with fecal material and cannot "see."

Perhaps the pill endoscopy will be feasible for viewing the colon one day, but this won't occur in the near future.

SCREENING SAVES LIVES

Recently, I treated a woman named Gabby, who had just turned fifty and was referred to me by her doctor for a colonoscopy. She was feeling healthy and fit, with absolutely no symptoms or signs of anything amiss in her digestive system. Nor did she have a family history of colon cancer, so she believed there was no cause for concern. But two of Gabby's friends had just been diagnosed with colon cancer, so she was highly motivated to undergo screening.

During her colonoscopy, I found a large polyp and removed it. Under microscopic evaluation, the polyp had high-grade dysplasia, meaning that it was one step away from turning into a full-blown cancer. Removing this polyp stopped the developing cancer, and colon cancer was nipped in the bud. Had she elected not to have this screening colonoscopy, or had she put it off, Gabby would have eventually developed a later-stage colon cancer that would have been more difficult to treat. Screening may have saved her life and she knows it! Let it save yours. The screening guidelines in tables 4-1A and 4-1B will help you identify exactly what you need to do.

Please don't put screening off. Please don't.

Table 4-1A

Colorectal Cancer Screening Guidelines for Men and Women at *Average* Risk

Average Risk Category

• Men and women at *average* risk (no symptoms or family history) for colorectal cancer should begin screening at age fifty years.

Screening Options

• Fecal occult blood testing (FOBT) once per year.
• Flexible sigmoidoscopy every 5 years.
• Combined (FOBT) with flexible sigmoidoscopy (FOBT every year, flexible sigmoidoscopy every 5 years)
• Colonoscopy every 10 years.
• Double contrast barium enema every 5 years.

Adapted from American Gastroenterological Association. 2003 (Winawer et al. *Gastroenterology* 2003; 124:544–560).

Table 4-1B

Colorectal Cancer Screening Guidelines for Men and Woman at *Increased* Risk

Family Risk Category	Screening Recommendation
• First-degree relative* affected with colorectal cancer or adenomatous polyp at age 60 or older.	Same as average risk, but start at age 40.

Family Risk Category	Screening Recommendation
• Two second-degree relatives† affected with colorectal cancer.	
• One first-degree relative with colorectal cancer or adenomatous polyps diagnosed younger than 60 years old.	Colonoscopy every 5 years starting at age 40 or 10 years younger than earliest diagnosis in the family, whichever comes first.
• Two or more first-degree relatives with colorectal cancer.	
• One second-degree or any third-degree** relative with colorectal cancer.	Same as average risk screening.

Hereditary (Inherited) Syndrome Risk Category	
• Gene carrier or family history of familial adenomatous polyposis (FAP).	Sigmoidoscopy annually, starting at age 10 to 12.
• Gene carrier or family history of hereditary nonpolyposis colorectal cancer (HNPCC).	Colonoscopy every 1 to 2 years, starting at age 20 to 25 or 10 years younger than earliest case in family, whichever comes first.

Personal Medical History Category	
• Personal history of inflammatory bowel disease (ulcerative colitis or Crohn's disease).	Colonoscopy with biopsy every 1 to 2 years, starting 7 to 8 years after diagnosis.
• Personal history of adenomatous polyps:	
• One or two small tubular adenomatous polyps (smaller than 1 cm).	First follow-up colonoscopy in 5 years.
• Advanced adenomatous polyps (1 cm or larger) or multiple polyps.	First follow-up colonoscopy in 3 years.
• Numerous polyps, polyp turned cancerous, or incomplete colonoscopy.	First follow-up colonoscopy at interval dependent on doctor's clinical judgment.
• Personal history of colorectal cancer:	
• Colon cancer and surgery to remove the cancer.	Colonoscopy at time of initial diagnosis to rule out other cancers and polyps.
• Colon cancer with obstruction before surgery.	Colonoscopy about 6 months after surgery to rule out other cancers and polyps.
	If colonoscopy after surgery is normal, a subsequent follow-up colonoscopy after 3 years. If normal, every 5 years thereafter.

*First-degree relative is a blood-related parent, sibling, or child.
†Second-degree relative is a grandparent, aunt, or uncle.
**Third-degree relative is a great-grandparent or cousin.

Adapted from: American Gastroenterological Association 2003 (Winawer et al. *Gastroenterology* 2003;124:544–560).

Chapter 5

Eat Smart, Live Right

In addition to regular screening, there is another important way for you to reduce your risk for developing colorectal cancer. You can do this by making simple adjustments to your lifestyle, such as eating a nutritious diet, staying physically fit, and avoiding harmful substances like alcohol and tobacco. These critical preventive measures are the subject of this chapter.

As I've looked into the medical evidence and employed it in my own practice, it has become more and more apparent to me that nutrition, exercise, and other positive lifestyle habits make a difference. For too many years, neither medicine nor doctors have thought enough about prevention and keeping people healthy. Although the power of medicine to fix problems after they have developed is immensely important, medicine's real power lies in the prevention of disease.

Most of the time, your doctor will tell you little or nothing about nutrition, supplements, or exercise, even though all of these may play a significant role in preventing many major diseases, including colorectal cancer. That's because until only very recently, these topics have simply not been a part of medical school curricula. Doctors had very little training in diet, nutrition, exercise, and other ways to prevent illness.

Doctors aren't entirely to blame for relegating prevention to a minor role in medicine, however. Many patients shoulder the blame as well. Think about it: Maybe you get a flu shot every year to protect yourself against the flu virus. Maybe you or your kids have been vaccinated against some obvious illness. But when was the last time you looked at oranges, apples, carrots, or spinach as medicines that could "inoculate" you against some life-threatening disease? What good does it do to have open-heart surgery if you just continue to eat artery-clogging fatty foods, or to be cured of colorectal cancer only to eat red meat every night for dinner? While miraculous medical technology and procedures can add years to our lives, most of us have enough bad habits to subtract the same number of years.

Many patients simply do not think about prevention, and they visit a doctor only when something is wrong. I often start off a new-patient visit by asking, "How can I help you today?" Most patients begin by describing what's bothering them. Only once did a patient say to me, "I feel fine, but you can help me by keeping me well." So you see, all of us, doctors and patients, must take a preventive approach to healing in order to improve our health, longevity, and quality of life.

Colorectal cancer can be lifestyle-related, so prevention is largely up to you, working in concert with your doctor. My hope is that you will get excited about what you learn here, and that you'll use this knowledge to help prevent colorectal cancer, or its recurrence, and live better—and longer.

COLON-FRIENDLY NUTRITION

At the Monahan Center, a common question I get from patients is: "What can I eat so that I will not get colorectal cancer?"

What I recommend to them is what I recommend to you: an eating plan that is low in fat (less than 30 percent of your total daily calories) and high in fiber (25 to 30 grams per day). It should be rich in fruits and vegetables, whole grains, beans and legumes, and lean proteins. It is a plan that you and your family can stick with for the rest of your life.

This approach to eating, incidentally, will help you lose weight if you need to. This is important, since obesity may be a risk factor for colorectal cancer.

A good example is Jamie, a healthy fifty-five-year-old woman with a family history of polyps. When she came to see me, she was about eighteen pounds overweight and really wanted to lose these excess pounds. At the same time, she was quite motivated to help prevent colorectal cancer, so she decided to follow my nutritional suggestions. She lost weight steadily, and as usually happens, friends began asking her, "What kind of diet are you on?" She simply told them she wasn't on a diet, but was following a healthy eating plan, with enough variety that she could eat foods she enjoyed.

Before I explain the substance of this plan, let's find out where you are right now in terms of your own nutritional habits. When you recognize areas needing attention, hopefully you'll become more motivated to changing them.

HOW COLON-FRIENDLY IS YOUR DIET?
TAKE THIS QUIZ TO FIND OUT

The following ten-question quiz is designed to give you a snapshot of problem areas in your diet. Answer each question with a simple yes or no, and be honest when responding so that you can see where you stand right now. Don't worry; no one is looking over your shoulder to grade you.

1. Do you eat red meat (beef, pork, lamb, or processed meats such as bacon, luncheon meats, sausage, hot dogs, or salami) once a week or less?
Yes__ No__

2. Do you eat two or more servings of nonfat or low-fat foods that are rich in calcium (such as milk, yogurt, or cheese) each day, or take 1,000 to 1,200 milligrams of supplemental calcium daily?
Yes__ No__

3. Do you take a multivitamin/mineral tablet most days of the week?
Yes__ No__

4. Do you drink, on average, less than one alcoholic beverage a day, or none at all?
Yes__ No__

5. Do you eat two to four servings of fruit each day?
Yes__ No__

6. Do you generally limit high-sugar, high-calorie foods (such as pie, cake, candy, chocolate, cookies, soda, or ice cream) in your diet?
Yes__ No__

7. Through the week, do you regularly choose high-fiber whole-grain carbohydrates (such as bran flakes, whole wheat bread or pasta, brown rice, or barley)?
Yes__ No__

8. Do you eat three to five servings of vegetables each day?
Yes__ No__

9. When you use fat or oil for food preparation, do you usually use olive oil, canola oil, or trans fat-free margarines?
Yes__ No__

10. Do you drink eight to ten cups of noncaffeinated fluid each day?
Yes__ No__

How Did You Do?

Tally up the number of your yeses, and interpret your score according to the following key:

• **9–10:** Congratulations. Your dietary habits are excellent and will go a long way toward helping prevent colorectal cancer.

• **6–8:** Good job. A score in this range indicates that you are doing a number of beneficial things. Review your no responses—

these are the weak spots in your efforts. Try to think of some changes you might make to turn your nos into yeses.

• **3–5:** A fair effort, but you can do better. The information in this chapter, and in the next, will put you on the road to better colon health.

• **0–2:** You may want to schedule an appointment with a registered dietician to help you plan a better nutritional program. It will be important for you to read this chapter and the next carefully, and begin to pay closer attention to your diet.

FOOD FOR THOUGHT

Foods have the remarkable power not only to nourish and energize us but also to help us stay fit. Eating right is thus one of the cornerstones to preventing colorectal cancer. What follows are the seven guiding principles that form the basis of my colon-friendly eating plan.

Principle 1: Take Advantage of the Healing Power of Fruits and Vegetables

Your mother was certainly right when she told you, "Eat your vegetables; they're good for you." Fruits and vegetables are loaded with nutrients that may help protect you from a number of chronic diseases, including colorectal cancer.

These natural anticancer agents include vitamins, minerals, and natural chemicals with hard-to-pronounce names such as *isothiocynates* or *saponins.* These plant chemicals, or phytochemicals, appear to have many important cancer-preventing functions.

Why are they protective? Phytochemicals, along with vitamins and minerals, have the ability to neutralize or scavenge free radicals—by-products of normal chemical reactions in your body that can make a cell turn malignant if not destroyed. These nutrients have other duties as well: They inhibit the formation of carcinogens (cancer-causing agents), bind carcinogens in the digestive tract and usher them out of the body, and provide the raw material in order to synthesize other anticancer agents in your body. They may also activate protective genes in your body.

Principle 2: Increase Fiber for Good Overall Digestive Health

Here we come to a nutrition topic that is simmering with controversy. For decades, it was a widely held belief in the medical and scientific community that fiber—the indigestible portion of food—would prevent colorectal cancer. And indeed, epidemiology studies, in which scientists look at a disease and try to figure out why one group of people has it or doesn't have it, have reported that populations with low-fiber diets have higher rates of colorectal cancer.

Then a study published in the prestigious *New England Journal of Medicine* in 2000 announced that fiber doesn't lower your risk of developing colorectal cancer at all. The researchers based their conclusions on an analysis of data from the ongoing Nurses' Health Study. In terms of protection against colorectal cancer, nurses who ate the most fiber (around twenty-five grams a day) were no better off, prevention-wise, than the women who ate only ten grams a day. The risk of cancer was the same, regardless of how much fiber was consumed.

The case for or against fiber is far from closed. New research has revived the notion that a high-fiber diet may protect against colorectal cancer. Two separate and independent studies—one based in the United States (The Prostate, Lung, Colorectal, and Ovarian Cancer Screening Trial, or PLCO) and one based in Europe (The European Prospective Investigation into Cancer and Nutrition, or EPIC)—associated high intake of dietary fiber with a decreased risk of either colonic adenomas or colorectal cancer. In the U.S. study, those in the highest fiber group, consuming thirty-six grams per day, had a twenty-seven percent lower risk of precancerous growths than those who ate the least (twelve grams a day). In the European study—the largest one ever conducted on cancer and nutrition—those who ate the highest amount of fiber (thirty-five grams a day) had about a forty percent lower risk of colorectal cancer compared with those who ate the least (about fifteen grams).

Why all the discrepancies? No one knows for sure. But quite possibly the source of fiber was different from study to study. Without getting too technical, fiber is actually a complex substance, with many different constituents. Fiber in fruits, for example, is a little different from fiber in grains. One type of fiber may do a better job of preventing colorectal cancer than another. Rather than debate the merits of various scientific studies, let me just emphasize that fiber is a very important nutrient for digestive health. If you eat a variety of fruits, vegetables, and whole grains, you'll get a well-rounded dose of all types of fiber.

Despite the controversy swirling around fiber, medical experts postulate this: Eating enough fiber helps reduce from your system a possible cancer promoter—bile acids. When fat and cholesterol are metabolized in your liver, bile acids are the by-product. Some bile acids may cause cells in the colon lining to proliferate; this *may* lead to the development of polyps and tumors.

Certain cereal fibers, namely wheat bran, dilute these bile acids, block their cancer-forming potential, and aid in excreting them from the body. You can reduce the formation of bile acids in other ways, too. Eating a low-fat and low-cholesterol diet also discourages the concentration of bile acids in your system and may even help lower your cholesterol. So does eating a diet rich in low-fat dairy products.

Fiber has other anticancer properties. It may activate a tumor suppressor gene to protect against abnormal cell growth. It speeds the passage of stool through your colon, thereby reducing its exposure to potential carcinogens. And fiber is digested by friendly bacteria in your colon—an action that may keep the colon lining healthy.

Fiber just makes good health sense—for other reasons as well. It helps in weight management and in the control of type 2 diabetes. It aids in protecting against heart disease. It puts an end to constipation and keeps you more regular. It relieves hemorrhoids and may improve other bowel problems such as irritable bowel syndrome and diarrhea. And it may prevent diverticulosis, a disease in which balloonlike pouches called diverticula form in the colon wall, usually a result of long-term constipation and low-fiber eating. Fiber can also help prevent the formation of new diverticula if you already have diverticulosis.

My Recommendation

Follow a high-fiber diet, which consists of between twenty-five and thirty-five grams of fiber a day or more. If you haven't been doing this, go easy at first. Gradually increase your fiber intake day by day, or else you'll suffer from bloating and gas and be asked to go to another room to eat your high-fiber meals. Try to drink eight to ten cups of fluid each day to avoid constipation. Include a variety of fiber-rich foods in your diet: whole grains, cereals, high-fiber breads, whole grain pasta, legumes (beans, peas, and lentils), and vegetables. Always choose fresh fruits instead of juice. Some of the best sources of fiber are listed in table 5-2. You can use this table as a guideline to help you make healthy choices.

Table 5-2

Fiber Sources

Grams of Fiber	Food Source
2–3 grams	**Fruits:** Apple with skin, 1 small Avocado (California), ¼ medium Banana, 1 medium Orange, 1 medium
	Vegetables: Cabbage, 1 cup raw, shredded Carrots, 1 medium raw Cauliflower, 1 cup cooked Spinach, 1 cup raw
	Breads: Bran bread (Branola) Whole wheat or rye, 1 slice Whole wheat English muffin, 1 whole
	Cereals: Post Shredded Wheat, General Mills Total or Wheaties, 1 cup Oatmeal, 1 packet Quaker Instant, or ¾ cup plain
	Grains: Barley, ½ cup Bulgur wheat, ⅓ cup
	Nuts: Almonds, sliced, ¼ cup
	Pasta: Whole wheat, ½ cup
	Rice: Brown rice, ½ cup Wild rice, ¼ cup
4–5 grams	**Fruits:** Dates, ¼ cup Pear with skin, 1 medium Prunes, 8 dried Raspberries, ½ cup Strawberries or blueberries, 1 cup
	Vegetables: Baked potato with skin, 1 small Sweet potato with skin, 1 medium Broccoli, cooked, 1 cup Brussels sprouts, frozen, boiled, 1 cup Corn, ½ cup or 1 ear

Grams of Fiber	Food Source
	Cereals: Post Grape-Nuts, ½ cup
	Kashi Heart to Heart, Kellogg's Raisin Bran, General Mills Bran Chex, or Post Bran Flakes, ¾ cup
	Popcorn, 3 cups
6 grams	Chickpeas, ½ cup
	Lentils, ½ cup
	Lima beans, ½ cup
8 grams or more	**Cereals:** Kellpgg's All-Bran, General Mills Fiber One, ½ cup
	Kashi Good Friends, ¾ cup
	Canned or cooked dried beans, ½ cup
	Figs (dried), 3
	Kidney beans, red, canned, ½ cup

Principle 3: Reduce Red Meat

You need a certain amount of protein from food to furnish the building material for your body and its many tissues, but one type of protein you don't need too much of is red meat, and this includes beef, pork, veal, and lamb. A lot of red meat in your diet is considered a risk factor for colorectal cancer.

Exactly why red meat is linked adversely to colorectal cancer is unknown at this time, but there are some theories. First, red meat is fatty, and fat steps up the production of bile acid, which may be harmful to colon cells. When cells are put in this bile acid–rich environment, they can start proliferating in an abnormal manner and may develop into polyps or cancer.

Second, red meat is high in iron, a characteristic that is both a blessing and a curse. The blessing: You need iron in your diet to build two critical proteins, hemoglobin and myoglobin. Hemoglobin is the oxygen-carrying component in your red blood cells, and myoglobin increases the supply of oxygen to your muscles to aid in physical movement.

The curse: Iron, unfortunately, is not well absorbed by your small intestine. The result is a potential buildup of iron in your colon. This accumulation sets in motion an unhealthy reaction in your colon referred to as oxidative stress; it occurs when free radicals, generated by excess iron, outnumber protective antioxidants. This situation may result in less-than-full protection against free radicals and may prevent your immune system from operating properly.

Finally, cooking meat generates two types of substances that are potential carcinogens: heterocyclic amines (HAs) and polycyclic aromatic hydrocarbons (PAHs).

HAs form in meat when you cook it at very high temperatures or beyond the just-done stage. Meat and poultry produce the most HAs because they contain a lot of protein substances that are converted into HAs when cooked. Charring the surface of the meat increases HAs. Fish produces much less HAs, and plant foods produce little or none.

PAHs are produced when fat drips down onto a heat source. They rise up in the smoke and land back on the food. They can also form directly on food when it's cooked to a crisp. HAs and PAHs that come in contact with the colon and rectal linings during digestion may promote cancer.

To reduce the formation of these substances in meat:

- Bake, roast, steam, or stew your meat. Other methods of cooking such as grilling, barbecuing, broiling, and pan-frying produce more HAs because these methods generate higher heat.
- Have your meat prepared medium rare, rather than well done.
- Do not eat blackened or charred food.
- If you love to grill, marinate your meat first for at least four hours; this eliminates most of the HAs that are produced.

My Recommendation

I'm not calling for the extinction of red meat in your diet. I do, however, recommend that you eat it only occasionally, maybe a few times a month. Select leaner cuts of meat, too. Examples include tenderloin, sirloin, eye of round, or top round.

Try grilling veggie burgers instead of hamburger patties. Make the switch to more fish in order to obtain the protein your body needs for growth and repair. Fish oil may even decrease your risk of colorectal cancer, according to research (see section on fat, below).

Principle 4: Go Easy on Fat

If there is one thing that cancer research is making clear, it is that higher intakes of saturated fat (found in meat, butter, and animal products), as well as trans fats (found in margarine, vegetable short-ening, and many commercially baked foods) may increase the risk of colorectal cancer.

Where saturated fat is concerned, researchers at the University of Texas Southwestern Medical Center suggest that the link to colorec-tal cancer may be partly due to the body's inability to cope with a buildup of lithocholic acid. This is a bile acid released by the body into the small intestine to help break down cholesterol. With a high-fat diet, where cholesterol is naturally abundant, more of this bile acid is produced than the body can handle. Lithocholic acid then makes its way through the intestine to the colon. It is thought that the high concentrations of this bile acid in the colon may lead to cancer.

A high intake of trans fats, also known as partially hydrogenated oils, makes conditions favorable for colorectal cancer, too, according to a University of Utah study, which analyzed the diets of more than four thousand men and women. These fats are created when liquid vegetable oils are synthetically altered through a process called hy-drogenation to make them solid. They are found in margarine, veg-etable shortening, and many commercially baked products. As to why trans fats increase risk, the investigators chalked it up to a num-ber of factors. Trans fats are known to compromise immunity; they also harm cell membranes, making it easy for cell damage to occur. These fats also appear to stimulate the activity of two enzymes, COX-1 and COX-2, which may be linked to tumor development in colorectal cancer. (I'll discuss these enzymes in more detail in the next chapter.)

What about the so-called good fats—monounsaturated fats and the omega-3s? Can you eat those? Absolutely.

One of the monounsaturated fats that may be protective against colorectal cancer is olive oil. Scientists have long observed that peo-ple in Mediterranean countries have very low rates of colorectal can-cer. A higher intake of olive oil has been singled out as one of the possible explanations. Olive oil contains a vitamin-like chemical called squalene, which has been shown to inhibit colon, lung, and skin tumors in rodents. Squalene is believed to work by suppressing an enzyme required for the growth of cancer cells. To date, no human studies have been conducted on the anticancer effect of squalene, although some investigators believe that it may turn out to be the key cancer fighter in olive oil.

One of the best ways to get the protective effects of good fats is to eat more fish, especially cold-water, fatty fish and shellfish—namely salmon, tuna, herring, sardines, rainbow trout, and oysters. The oil in these species of fish and shellfish contains what are commonly known as omega-3 fats. There is a fair body of research showing that these healthy fats may decrease the abnormal growth of cells in the lining of the colon.

My Recommendation

Keep your fat intake to within 30 percent of your daily calories. Saturated fat intake should be less than 10 percent of your total calories. If you don't want to do any bothersome calculations or arithmetic, here are some tips that will help you automatically slash your fat intake:

- Emphasize mostly plant foods, as well as lean poultry (without the skin) and fish in your diet.
- Consume at least three servings of omega-3-rich fish per week.
- Cut back on your use of butter and margarine, as well as mayonnaise, regular-fat salad dressings, and fried foods.
- Substitute olive or canola oil for corn or safflower oil in your cooking, and add a handful of nuts to your yogurt or chunks of avocado to your salad.
- Use low-fat or fat-free salad dressings, instead of regular-fat dressings.
- Reduce your intake of packaged or processed foods such as frozen dinners, cakes, cookies, chips, and fast-food items (pizza, doughnuts, cheeseburgers, and fries). These foods are usually high in saturated fats and trans fats.

Principle 5: Dairy—Milk It for All It's Worth

Low-fat dairy products, such as skim or 1 percent milk, low-fat or nonfat yogurt, and low-fat cheeses, are rich sources of a number of anticancer substances:

• **Calcium,** a mineral that protects against colorectal cancer. (You'll be hearing more from me about calcium in the next chapter.)

• **Vitamin D,** another nutrient that protects against colorectal cancer. (I'll talk about vitamin D in the next chapter, too.)

• **Conjugated linoleic acid (CLA),** a beneficial fat that acts as an antioxidant and has been shown to inhibit colon cancer in lab animals. Low-fat milk is a good source of CLA.

• **Probiotics,** friendly bacteria that are found in yogurt and other fermented dairy products. Probiotics prevent disease-causing bacterial intruders from multiplying and doing harm. Though more research is needed, probiotics (in yogurt) have been linked to a reduced risk of colon cancer and improved immunity in lab animals.

MY RECOMMENDATION

Each day, you should aim for at least two to three servings of low-fat or skim milk, reduced-fat sugar-free yogurt, or reduced-fat cheese. A serving consists of one cup of milk or yogurt, or two ounces of reduced-fat cheese. If you are lactose intolerant (lactose is the natural sugar found in milk), try to find lactose-reduced or lactose-free dairy substitute.

Principle 6: De-sugar Your Diet

Too much sugar and too many sugar-containing foods in your diet may be linked to an increased risk of colon cancer. In one large-scale study, the Iowa Women's Health Study, investigators found that the risk of colon cancer increased twofold in women whose diets were high in sugar and foods to which sugar was added. Other studies involving both men and women have reported similar findings.

So it's wise to make de-sugaring your diet a priority. When I say *de-sugar,* I'm referring to added sugar—found mostly in what we call junk food or sweet treats. Added sugar may play a role in a huge host of health problems, including obesity, diabetes, heart disease, and cancer.

The mystery by which added sugar increases risk hasn't been entirely solved yet, but some credible theories have been advanced. First, researchers believe that added sugar slows down the movement of food through your gastrointestinal tract, thereby increasing the time carcinogens are exposed to tissue. Second, added sugar increases your system's concentration of bile acids (the possible cancer promoters I have been talking about). And third, an excess of added sugar over the long term may upset your body's normal production of the hormone insulin, and this may stimulate abnormal cell division.

MY RECOMMENDATION

- Cut back on desserts, candy, cookies, baked goods, presweetened cereals, soft drinks, fruit beverages, jams, fruited yogurt, cakes, and any food products that list sugar as one of their first few ingredients.
- Start reading food labels more carefully. Try to select food items that contain less than 30 grams of total carbohydrate (not just sugar because carbohydrates break down into sugar during digestion). Look for words ending in *–ose,* since these indicate the presence of added sugars. Additives such as corn syrup and high-fructose corn syrup count as added sugar, too.
- Avoid drinking your sugars. This includes sodas, fruit drinks, sweetened iced teas, and "ades" like lemonade.

Principle 7: Water Your Digestive System

An essential but often overlooked nutrient is water. Our bodies are 60 percent water, and it is required for growth, development, and overall health. Among many other vital functions, water is the medium of transport for nutrients and waste products in your body.

If you're following the high-fiber approach to eating that I emphasized earlier, you should drink well beyond the call of thirst. Fiber requires the presence of water for proper processing in your digestive system and works together with water and other fluids to create larger, softer stools. Without enough water, fiber acts like a chunk of cement—and moves through your system about as fast. Too little water in a high-fiber diet many cause dehydration and lead to the very condition fiber is meant to prevent: constipation.

If your body is consistently water-deficient—that is, you just don't drink enough water on a regular basis—increasing your water intake may make you feel more energetic and perhaps reduce your risk of colon cancer. Several years ago, researchers at the Fred Hutchinson Cancer Research Center, Seattle, conducted a study of the relationship between diet and colon cancer. When the data from a diet questionnaire completed by more than four hundred men and women with a history of colon cancer were analyzed, an unexpected finding emerged. Among women who drank more than five glasses of plain water a day, there was a reduced incidence of colon cancer. Men who drank more than four glasses of water a day had fewer cases of colon cancer. This is not the only study to suggest a benefit of water drinking; a couple of other studies have found a link between high intake of water and reduced risk of colon and rectal cancers.

Although water appears to be beneficial to colon health, scientists aren't yet sure why. It may be that increased water intake helps prevent constipation and speeds up transit time of waste moving through the digestive system. This might minimize contact with cancer-causing agents in the colon and rectum.

My Recommendation

Drink eight to ten glasses of plain water a day, depending on the amount of fluid available from juices, tea, or coffee. If you're very active, you may need to bump your water intake up to over ten glasses a day. Try to drink water with every meal, as well as with snacks, and keep a water bottle close by to quench your thirst. For flavor and variety, try adding some slices of lemon, lime, or cucumbers; flavored seltzers are also a good choice.

I also suggest that you periodically check the color of your urine to assess whether you're drinking enough water. If the color is dark or the odor is strong, increase your intake. Light-colored urine is a good sign that you're well hydrated. Always treat your body as you would the plants in your garden—water it on a regular basis.

PREVENTIVE EATING

Now that you understand the basic principles of colon-friendly nutrition—high in plant foods and fiber; rich in calcium; low in fat,
red meat, and sugar; and sufficient in fluids—it's time to put it in
action. Table 5-3 below is a tool you can stick on your refrigerator
to remind you of what to eat each day. *You don't have to follow it exactly; it is only a guideline. Just do your best.* I've also provided three
sample menus that you may use as guidelines to assist you in your
own meal planning.

Table 5-3

Foods to Choose

Cereals, whole grains, and pastas: *Approximately six to eight servings daily*	Oatmeal, oat bran, All-Bran, 40% Bran, raisin bran, Multi-Bran Chex, and high-fiber cereal (3 or more grams of fiber per serving); Branola, whole wheat bread, cracked wheat bread, multigrain bread, pumpernickel or rye bread, bran muffins; brown rice; whole wheat pasta. (One serving equals 1 slice bread, 1 muffin, ¾ cup dry cereal, or ½ cup cooked cereal, rice, or pasta.)
High-fiber vegetables: *At least three to five servings from this group daily*	Raw vegetables, salad vegetables, cooked vegetables, green leafy vegetables. (One serving equals 1 cup raw vegetables or ½ cup cooked vegetables.) Look for variety and color.
Starchy vegetables: *One serving daily from this group*	Potatoes, sweet potatoes, winter squash, legumes (beans, lentils, or peas). (One serving equals 1 medium potato or ½ cup cooked squash or legumes. Legumes may be used as protein substitute.)
Fruit: *Two to four servings from this group daily*	Any fresh fruit, stewed fruit (especially figs, prunes, or apricots), dried fruit (especially figs, prunes, apricots, or raisins), canned or cooked fruit, any natural unsweetened fruit juice. (One serving equals 1 medium fruit, ½ cup stewed fruit, 4–6 pieces dried fruit, 2–3 tablespoons raisins, ½ cup canned or cooked fruit, 1 cup fruit juice.) Look for variety and color.
Dairy: *Two to three servings from this group daily*	Low-fat milk, skim milk, yogurt, soy milk, tofu, reduced-fat cheeses. (One serving equals 1 cup milk or yogurt, or ½ cup tofu, or 2 ounces reduced-fat cheese.)
Lean protein: *Three to four servings daily*	Poultry, fish, shellfish, and eggs. One serving of eggs equals one egg or two egg whites. (Limit eggs to no more than 4 per week if you are being treated for heart disease.)
Healthy fats: *One to two servings from this group daily*	Olive oil, flaxseed oil, canola oil, reduced-fat salad dressing, reduced-fat peanut butter, trans-fat-free margarines, unoiled nuts or seeds. (One serving equals 1 tablespoon oil, trans-fat-free margarines, reduced-fat peanut butter, nuts, or seeds; or 2 tablespoons reduced-fat salad dressing.)

Foods to Choose (continued)

Condiments	Salt, sugar substitutes, fat-free salad dressings, catsup, tomato sauce, wheat bran, herbs, spices.

Foods to Avoid or Use Sparingly

Red meat, white bread, cakes, sweets, pastries and biscuits, chocolate, sodas, and alcohol.

SAMPLE MEAL PLAN 1

Breakfast
Bowl of Multi-Bran Chex, ¾ cup
1 cup fresh strawberries
1 cup skim or 1 percent milk
Water, coffee, or tea

Snack
½ cup 1 percent cottage cheese with ½ banana

Lunch
Big bowl of mixed dark field greens (such as romaine lettuce) tossed with chunks of tomato, cucumber, carrots, ¼ cup white beans, and ¼ cup cannellini beans
2 tablespoons nonfat raspberry vinaigrette dressing on the side for dipping
Water or sugar-free beverage

Snack
¼ cup mixed nuts (almonds, walnuts, pecans), with ¼ cup mixed dried fruit (apricots, pears, cranberries, apples)
Water

Dinner
4–6 ounces grilled salmon
½ cup quinoa
1 cup steamed asparagus (with olive oil)
Tossed salad with nonfat dressing
Water or sugar-free beverage

SAMPLE MEAL PLAN 2

Breakfast
1 cup low-fat plain yogurt, with mixed berries: ½ cup raspberries, ¼ cup blueberries, and ¼ cup blackberries
Water, coffee, or tea

Snack
1 whole wheat English muffin, toasted, with 1 tablespoon reduced-fat peanut butter
Water

Lunch
1 cup lentil soup
½ sandwich or wrap (grilled chicken, turkey, or vegetables)
1 medium-size plum
Water or sugar-free beverage

Snack
⅓ cup hummus, with 1 cup fresh crunchy veggie sticks (cut-up pepper, zucchini, baby carrots, cherry tomatoes)

Dinner
4-ounce chicken breast, sautéed with mixed vegetables (broccoli, carrots, pea pods, and water chestnuts) in canola oil with reduced-sodium soy sauce
⅔ cup brown rice
Water or sugar-free beverage

SAMPLE MEAL PLAN 3

Breakfast
Omelet: 2 egg whites, mixed with 1 cup vegetables (such as spinach and mushrooms) and 2 ounces part-skim mozzarella cheese
1 slice whole wheat bread, toasted, with Smart Beat margarine (trans-fat-free)
Water, coffee, or tea

Snack

1 low-fat bran or blueberry muffin
1 cup skim or low-fat milk (or soy milk)

Lunch

Whole wheat pita bread, stuffed with tuna (water-packed, mixed with nonfat mayonnaise) and cut-up veggies (romaine lettuce, tomatoes, shredded carrots, bean sprouts)
1 orange
Water or sugar-free beverage

Snack

1 cup nonfat yogurt sprinkled with ¼ cup low-fat granola or ¼ cup Grape-Nuts cereal

Dinner

1 cup vegetarian bean chili
6 whole wheat crackers or rye crisp bread
Tossed salad with nonfat dressing
Water or sugar-free beverage

LIVE RIGHT

Eating smart goes a long way toward prevention and good health. But so do other lifestyle habits, namely being physically active, curbing your alcohol use, and quitting smoking. All three lifestyle factors can help reduce your risk of colorectal cancer. Let's take a closer look.

EXERCISE: A VITAL STEP TO PREVENTION

Exercise has proven to be an unexpected friend in the fight against colorectal cancer. The Nurses' Health Study, for example, found that exercise slashes a woman's risk of developing colon cancer and adenomatous polyps in half. Other scientific investigations have found similar benefits for men.

How can being physically fit prevent colorectal cancer? Nobody knows for sure, but there are several possible explanations. One reason exercise may protect you is because it stimulates the motility of your colon, shortening the time and exposure that potential cancer-promoting materials remain in contact with its lining.

Other colorectal-cancer-preventing properties of exercise include: increasing the activity of antioxidants, which scavenge free radicals; enhancing your immune system; and reducing body fat (obesity raises the risk for colorectal cancer). On the other side of the equation, not exercising may raise your levels of insulin and insulin-like growth hormone, two chemicals that in excess are thought to stimulate cells in the colon to grow abnormally.

The big question is: How hard or how much should you exercise to ward off colorectal cancer? In studies so far, moderate activity seems to work as well as very intense exercise. The Nurses' Health Study researchers noted that walking at a normal to brisk pace (that's about three miles per hour) for one hour provided as much protection against colon cancer as jogging, bicycling, or swimming for half an hour a day. Considering the evidence researchers have compiled on exercise as a preventive measure, a good, overall recommendation is to log in at least thirty minutes a day in order to lower your risk of colorectal cancer.

Almost any type of physical activity works well for the prevention of colorectal cancer, so rather than give you a specific prescription for what to do, I will give you some easy ways to sneak exercise into your life.

The good news is that you don't have to work out in a gym or engage in a structured exercise program—unless you want to. There is compelling scientific proof that simple lifestyle activity can truly provide benefits similar to traditional workouts. A powerful case in point: In a Johns Hopkins University study, forty overweight women were instructed to either follow a step aerobics program three times a week for sixteen weeks or increase their daily lifestyle activity by thirty minutes a day most days of the week. Both groups followed a low-fat twelve-hundred calorie-a-day diet. By the end of the experimental period, all the women had lost nearly the same amount of weight; eighteen pounds in the aerobics group and seventeen pounds in the lifestyle group. The two groups also showed comparable improvements in important health measures such as blood pressure, cholesterol and triglycerides profiles, and overall cardiovascular fitness. This study suggests to me that increased lifestyle activity, plus a low-fat diet, can be just as effective for increasing fitness levels as a structured aerobics exercise program. That's great news if you have trouble fitting structured exercise into your schedule.

Even on-the-job activity counts. When I meet with patients for the first time and get to know them, I usually ask, "What do you do for a living?" If they tell me they are construction workers, carpenters, mail carriers, furniture movers, or employees in other jobs requiring physical labor, that's positive news in terms of on-the-job exercise and colorectal cancer risk reduction.

How, then, can you begin to integrate physical activity into your life? The first step is to give some thought to your daily routine and plan ways to work in more activity. Check with your doctor first to make sure you are medically able to tolerate increased physical activity. Here are some suggestions:

- Try taking the stairs more often, rather than the elevator or escalator. Stair climbing is a great way to enhance your cardiovascular fitness and to improve your leg strength, because you'll be lifting your body against gravity.
- Assess your environment: Can you stop using the closest vending machine, coffee station, restroom, or parking space? Set your life up so that you walk the longest route to wherever you're headed.
- Do your own housework. Play some music while you work, making it fun, and move your body to the rhythm of the music. You'll burn up about 250 calories an hour; more (450) if you scrub floors for an hour.
- Do gardening and yard work. Though not as aerobic as running, both activities provide the same fitness benefits as a steady walk. Planting, weeding, digging, and other forms of gardening expend roughly 220 calories in an hour.
- Become a do-it-yourselfer. Painting, hanging wallpaper, and doing light carpentry provide the same metabolic results as a brisk walk.

- If you take a subway, train, taxi, or bus to your place of employment, get off a stop or two earlier and walk the rest of the way.
- Pursue a new sport. Playing sports is fun, and you'd be surprised at how many calories you'll burn up in just an hour. Sports, such as basketball, tennis, bowling, golf (carrying your own bag), and badminton use up between 300 and 450 calories an hour—even more than a brisk walk!

No matter what activity or activities you choose, try to get in at least half an hour of lifestyle activity each day. You can accrue your thirty minutes, too—ten minutes here, ten minutes there—as opposed to setting aside a formal half-hour exercise session each day. Just make sure to pick an activity you enjoy!

CURB YOUR ALCOHOL INTAKE

Alcoholism is a worldwide epidemic. I am stunned at how many individuals I incidentally discover with this disease—and, trust me, it is a disease. The worst part about alcoholism is the denial. Alcohol abuse may be crystal clear to everybody else in the world, but unless the individual recognizes his or her addiction, that person will never be able to get help. Without help, alcoholism is as deadly as the most advanced case of colon cancer. I mention this because alcohol consumption is also a risk factor for colorectal cancer.

What I seek to do in my practice is identify patients who may have a history of drinking-related problems or be alcoholics and not realize it. That way, I can appropriately counsel them on the potential dangers of alcohol abuse and the best course of action. The approach that I use when I take health histories is called CAGE, a series of four questions designed to evaluate alcohol use:

*C*ut: Have you ever felt that you should cut down on your drinking?

*A*nnoyed: Have you ever become annoyed by criticism of your drinking?

*G*uilt: Have you ever felt guilty about your drinking?

*E*ye-opener: Have you ever had a morning eye-opener to get rid of a hangover?

If you answered yes to one question, it indicates that you quite possibly are an alcohol abuser; if you answered yes to more than one, it indicates probable alcoholism. In either case, talk to your family doctor about enrolling in an appropriate treatment program for alcohol problems.

On the other hand, if you are a social drinker, remember that even moderate drinking (one glass of wine, one can of beer, one mixed drink, or one shot of hard alcohol a day) may increase your risk of colorectal cancer, although some studies say it is beneficial for your heart. If you believe this, think about your colon and the rest of your body before you use alcohol for medicinal purposes.

PUT OUT CIGARETTES

As I discussed earlier in the book, people with a long history of smoking are at a greater risk of colorectal cancer. So if you thought I was harsh on alcohol, just wait until you hear what I have to say about smoking. I think I can summarize it this way: Tobacco is harmful to every organ system in the body and causes more disease, suffering, and premature death than any other known legal substance out there—period.

If you're a smoker, talk to your doctor about some of the new methods for quitting that may be appropriate for you, such as:

- Medications like Zyban
- Nicotine gum
- Nicotine patches
- Nicotine inhalers
- Smoking-cessation programs

The information I have shared with you here doesn't guarantee that diet, exercise, and other lifestyle habits will prevent you from getting colorectal cancer, but they do pay large health dividends. The evidence strongly suggests that people who follow healthy diets and are physically active are less likely to get colorectal cancer. So you want to be sure you're a member of the crowd who eats a healthy diet, stays fit through exercise, and enjoys the protective, revitalizing benefits that flow from a healthy lifestyle.

Chapter 6

Curb Colorectal Cancer:
Supplements and Chemoprevention

How many times have you heard that there is some special vitamin, mineral, or herb that can prevent cancer? This is a topic of immense interest, since cancer will touch every one of our lives in one way or another. Wouldn't it be nice if there were something simple you could take that would eliminate your chances of getting cancer?

Unfortunately, life is not this simple, and while I do believe in supplementation, I do not believe that there is a single magical agent that can prevent cancer. There are some who claim unequivocally that certain agents will stop cancer-triggering processes; others, staunch traditionalists, will insist that no vitamin, mineral, herb, or drug could possibly prevent cancer. Separating fact from fiction isn't easy, and doctors, who are inundated with material, simply don't have time to sift through every piece of information on nutrients for which there is a disease-preventing claim. Moreover, most "cancer preventing" claims are made with limited data that are published in remote journals. For these reasons, seldom will you get a thorough answer from your doctor, or even a recommendation, on what supplements you should take, and in what amounts.

In my own practice, I believe in offering the best of both conventional and complementary medicine. Supplementation and chemoprevention are a huge part of this approach. *Chemoprevention* refers to the use of medications and vitamin and mineral supplements to prevent, reverse, or suppress the progression of precancerous cells to full-blown cancer. (Don't confuse this term with the cancer treatment known as chemotherapy.)

I believe certain supplements and other agents work preventively if you've never had cancer and want to protect yourself. What's more, they are equally important if you're at increased risk, or you're a colorectal cancer survivor who wants to reduce the risk of recurrent cancer. Hopefully, more doctors will begin to practice medicine in this way as they learn about supplementation and chemoprevention.

In my own work, I have objectively sifted through and analyzed the scientific data for a number of nutrients and other agents for which anti-colon-cancer claims have been made, and I have concluded that seven agents show some promise in preventing colorectal cancer. They are:

- Folic acid
- Calcium
- Vitamin D
- Selenium
- Vitamin E
- Nonsteroidal anti-inflammatory drugs (NSAIDs)
- Hormone replacement therapy (HRT)

What follows is my analysis of each and my advice on how to use them in a sensible manner. *One precaution:* Never take supplements or other agents without consulting first with your physician.

POLYP-FIGHTING FOLIC ACID

Folic acid isn't an acid at all; it's a B vitamin that is essential for normal cell growth and healthy blood. Basically, folic acid helps your body synthesize the DNA required for new cells, and it is required for normal cell division. Technically speaking, *folate* is the form of the vitamin found naturally in foods, while *folic acid* refers to the form found in supplements. I'll use the term *folic acid*, since it is probably most familiar to you.

This is a very exciting time for folic acid. It has been found to play a role in preventing heart disease and neural tube defects (a disabling birth defect in newborns), and reducing the risk of certain cancers, including colorectal cancer. Its cancer-blocking benefits have only recently been discovered.

FOLIC ACID AND COLORECTAL CANCER

Researchers have linked low blood levels of folic acid with an increased risk of colorectal cancer and a high intake of folic acid (from food and multivitamin supplementation) with a decreased risk. One of the most impressive studies addressing folic acid and colon cancer is the famed Nurses' Health Study. This research discovered that nurses who took a multivitamin containing folic acid for at least fifteen years reduced their risk of colorectal cancer by as much as 75 percent compared to women who did not take vitamins; those who took multivitamins for between five and ten years reduced their risk by 20 percent. Folic acid is just as protective in men, according to other studies. It is important for me to add here that other research has found that folic acid may help regulate cell growth in patients with ulcerative colitis, an inflammatory bowel disease that is a known risk factor for colon cancer.

Exactly how folic acid acts as a risk reducer for colorectal cancer is unknown. Scientists suspect, however, that there may be at least three fundamental ways by which it works: It may decrease the likelihood of genetic mutations that lead to colon cancer, assist in the repair of damaged genes, or protect against errors when genes are copied during cell division. Any one of these actions could possibly likely stop or reverse precancerous conditions.

Best Food Sources

The name *folate* originates from the Latin word *folia*, "leaves." Accordingly, dark green leafy vegetables such as spinach, kale, and romaine lettuce are among the richest sources of folic acid. Other foods high in the substance include asparagus, broccoli, brussels sprouts, lima beans, peas, sweet potatoes, cantaloupe, oranges, orange juice, oatmeal, wheat germ, fortified grains and cereals, wild rice, and liver.

Your body cannot make folic acid; you have to get it from food or supplements. Eating foods rich in this vitamin helps ensure that you get an adequate supply. But for the greatest protection, supplement your diet with a basic multivitamin. (See below.)

Dosage: How Much Should You Take?

The amount of folic acid you normally need each day is 400 micrograms, the quantity available in virtually any brand of multivitamin supplement. Folic acid is safe when taken in dosages less than 1,000 micrograms a day. Exceeding the recommended dose can mask a vitamin B_{12} deficiency.

As to which supplement to choose, select a recognizable product manufactured by a well-known company. That way, you have the best chance of getting a quality supplement with a formulation that is true to its labeled ingredients.

Precautions

Of all vitamins, folic acid seems to have the most adverse interactions with certain prescription medications. Taking folic acid supplements may reduce the effectiveness of the following medications: methotrexate (Rheumatrex), colchicines (ColBenemid), trimethoprim (Trimpex, Bactrim, Septra), pyrimethamine (Daraprim, Fansidar), trimetrexate (NeuTrexin), and phenytoin (Dilantin). Folic acid may also interact adversely with certain chemotherapy agents. If you are taking any of these medications or undergoing chemotherapy, talk to your doctor about supplementing with folic acid.

Another important issue: Aspirin may interfere with your body's ability to use folic acid by changing the acid balance of your stomach so do not take aspirin and folic acid together. Instead, take one in the morning and one in the evening.

Finally, if you are at risk for pernicious anemia, a disease associated with a lack of stomach acid and poor absorption of vitamin B_{12}, use folic acid supplements only under your doctor's supervision. Risk factors for these conditions include a family history of the disease, as well as certain autoimmune diseases such as type 1 diabetes, hypoparathyroidism, Addison's disease, and Graves' disease.

CALCIUM FOR PREVENTION AND FOR THE POLYP-PRONE

The message that calcium builds bones and protects against osteoporosis (a bone-thinning disease) has been drummed into us a million times. But calcium's value as a benefactor in the human body goes far beyond bone health. Researchers have found that this well-known mineral plays a role in guarding against heart disease and many other major diseases, including colorectal cancer. Calcium has been shown in research to decrease the incidence of polyp formation and colorectal cancer.

Calcium and Colorectal Cancer

Calcium appears to have an inhibiting effect on colon cancer growth at the cellular level. One of the earliest investigations into this was conducted at Memorial Sloan-Kettering Cancer Center in 1985. There, researchers looked into what effect calcium supplements might have on the colon tissue of people with a strong family tendency to develop colon cancer. Before taking calcium supplements, these high-risk individuals had an unusually high rate of cell division in their colons. As part of the experiment, they supplemented with a dose of 1,250 milligrams of calcium a day. After two to three months of supplementation, their colon cells stopped dividing at the abnormally high rate and took on a rate of cell division more characteristic of people at a low risk of colon cancer.

Over the years, the calcium–colon cancer connection has grown stronger. One of the most interesting studies comes from St. Luke's–Roosevelt Hospital Center and Columbia University in New York City, where researchers studied people with a history of polyps. They found that increasing daily calcium intake by up to 1,200 milligrams from low-fat dairy products—rich sources of calcium—reduced the number of colon cells that foreshadowed early signs of cancer.

A team of researchers at Harvard School of Public Health strengthened the case for calcium when they borrowed data from the Nurses' Health Study and the Health Professionals Study—a total of more than 135,000 people—and analyzed the information for correlations between calcium and colon cancer. As it turned out, the risk of developing colon cancer in the distal (left side) colon was about 50 percent lower in those who consumed approximately 700 milligrams a day or more of calcium, compared to those who consumed 500 milligrams a day or less. The findings suggest that even a slight increase in your calcium intake may be protective against colon cancer.

How exactly does calcium work to possibly ward off colon cancer? No one knows with absolute certainty. But researchers theorize that in the colon, calcium latches onto bile and fatty acids and makes them insoluble so they can be excreted. When soluble, these substances can encourage cells to multiply uncontrollably. Calcium from both food and supplements seems to confer this protective benefit.

Best Food Sources

The richest dietary sources of calcium are dairy products. Other sources include spinach, collard greens, broccoli, and tofu, although much less calcium is absorbed from these foods than from dairy products. Almonds also have a good supply of calcium.

Dosage: How Much Should You Take?

The recommended daily intake for calcium is 1,000 milligrams a day if you're between the ages of nineteen and fifty; and 1,200 milligrams a day if you're older than fifty. Most adults get far less than the required amounts, making supplementation an excellent idea.

When it comes to colorectal cancer, however, taking only 700 to 800 milligrams a day seems to confer a benefit to men and women.

Increasing the dose beyond 800 milligrams does not appear to offer any additional protection.

For my male readers: Some worrisome data in the medical literature link calcium supplementation (dosages of 1,500 milligrams and higher) with an increased risk of prostate cancer. For this reason, I do not routinely recommend calcium supplementation for men unless they have a medical reason for it, such as osteoporosis.

Certainly, the full story on calcium as a colorectal cancer preventive agent has yet to be written, and a lot more research needs to be done before we figure out exactly what's going on. But based on what we do know, I believe in recommending increased calcium for women—first from food, and second from supplements, as a backup. Most women have already been told to increase their calcium intake to prevent osteoporosis. Therefore, my recommendation for women is just a reiteration of what they should already be doing.

Which Calcium Supplement Is Best?

I suggest the following guidelines to my patients:

- Try to get your calcium from food first. If following a calcium-rich diet is difficult for you, however, then taking a calcium supplement is a good idea.
- Take a calcium supplement that is either calcium carbonate or calcium citrate. Made from limestone, calcium carbonate is found in products such as Caltrate, Os-cal, and Tums. Calcium citrate is found in Citracal.
- Take your calcium supplement with a meal for better absorption. Calcium carbonate, in particular, requires stomach acid from the digestion of food for absorption. Consider spreading your dose throughout the day—your body can absorb only about 500 milligrams of calcium at a time. Taking calcium between meals is risky, since many calcium supplements, regardless of their calcium source, are not well absorbed without the presence of food.
- Avoid calcium supplements made from oyster shells; these

contain too much lead, which is toxic to the body. Labels don't usually specify the source as oyster shells, but if the product says "natural" calcium carbonate, then it's probably oyster-shell calcium. You see, in this case, *natural* does not necessarily mean "better." Calcium supplements made from bonemeal and dolomite also contain lead.

- Do not buy coral calcium, which has been falsely promoted as having anticancer properties beyond what calcium alone can do. No medical evidence supports this claim. Coral calcium contains limestone, the same calcium source found in calcium carbonate—but it may also contain lead. Further, coral calcium is roughly four times as expensive as regular store-brand calcium carbonate.

- With the exception of chewable and liquid products (which I recommend), some calcium products are not soluble enough to do any good; this is a prevailing problem with certain calcium supplements. You can do a simple test yourself at home to see whether your calcium supplement disintegrates well enough to be useful. Simply place the supplement in a cup of vinegar. If it disintegrates within half an hour, the supplement has sufficient dissolution.

Precautions

If you are under age sixty-five, there are very few side effects associated with calcium supplementation. In some people over age sixty-five, there may be mild side effects, and these include bloating and constipation.

If you are taking medications that reduce stomach acid, your body will not absorb calcium carbonate well. These include Pepcid, Zantac, Axid, Tagamet, Prilosec, Nexium, Prevacid, Aciphex, and Protonix. In such cases, a better alternative may be calcium citrate because it can be absorbed without the presence of stomach acid. Calcium citrate is also a good choice if you have a sensitive stomach.

In addition, some kidney stones are composed of calcium. If you have any history of kidney stones, or a condition known as hyperparathyroidism, you should speak to your doctor before taking calcium supplements.

THE VITAMIN D DEFENSE

Vitamin D helps your body absorb calcium and deposit it in your bones and teeth. If you're a woman who is postmenopausal and vulnerable to osteoporosis, you need an adequate supply of this vitamin. Vitamin D also has strong implications for preventing colorectal cancer.

Your most abundant supply of vitamin D is obtained directly from the sun. When a cholesterol derivative in your skin is hit by sunlight, a chemical change takes place—it turns into vitamin D and is absorbed into your bloodstream. If you get enough sunlight each day—roughly fifteen minutes of exposure—then you don't really have to worry too much about obtaining vitamin D from your diet. That amount of sunlight is enough to eliminate any need for dietary vitamin D if you're a healthy adult. That being said, I would not rely on sun exposure for your vitamin D requirements. Most people do not (and probably should not because of the risk of skin cancer) get this type of sun exposure.

Vitamin D and Colorectal Cancer

Research into vitamin D suggests strongly that the nutrient has an anticancer benefit. In a recent large study among thirteen VA medical centers, dietary vitamin D dominated calcium and folate as an important protective factor for large polyps and cancer. And research conducted by scientists in Spain, using human colon cancer cells cultured in lab dishes, revealed that vitamin D prevents runaway cell growth and converts cancerous cells into cells that appear more normal.

The exact mechanism by which vitamin D works in this way is not fully understood, but it may have something to do with how vitamin D and calcium interact. More research is needed on vitamin D, but the evidence compiled so far seems to indicate that getting adequate amounts of vitamin D is an important defense.

Best Food Sources

The best source of vitamin D is from the sun, but make sure you do not overdo, since excessive sun exposure carries its own risk of skin cancer including melanoma. Further, too much sun exposure can damage your skin, resulting in premature aging and wrinkling.

Food sources of vitamin D include fatty saltwater fish such as tuna, halibut, mackerel, herring, and sardines, as well as vitamin-D-fortified milk and enriched breakfast cereals. Maitake and shiitake mushrooms are also good sources. Many calcium supplements are formulated with vitamin D, and this is a good way to ensure that you are getting enough, especially if you are not in the sun very much.

Dosage: How Much Should You Take?

My recommendation is to supplement your diet with vitamin D. Based on guidelines for daily vitamin D requirements from the National Academy of Sciences, I advise a total vitamin D intake of 200 IUs daily if you are nineteen to fifty years old; 400 IUs daily if you are ages fifty-one to seventy; and 600 IUs daily if you are older than seventy.

OTHER SUPPLEMENTAL NUTRIENTS: SELENIUM

What can other vitamins and minerals do to fight polyps and prevent colon cancer? Possibly, quite a lot. Some nutrients to watch are selenium and vitamin E. There is less conclusive evidence on these two supplements, but I still believe they are worth considering.

Let's start with selenium, a mineral that functions as an antioxidant and repairs damage to cells. It helps manufacture a special enzyme, glutathione peroxidase, that turns peroxides (which are caustic to cell membranes) into harmless water. Selenium may also help prevent cancer by delaying cell division long enough for a damaged cell to repair its DNA.

Selenium and Colorectal Cancer

Most of the research into selenium and colorectal cancer has been conducted with animals, and it indicates that the mineral slows the growth of cancer. But we also know that colon cancer rates are high in regions where the selenium content of water and soil is deficient, and low in areas where there is a high selenium level. That's a clue as to selenium's potential protective effect against colon cancer. Still, the notion that selenium lowers the overall risk of cancer has not been firmly established.

Best Food Sources

The best food sources of selenium are Brazil nuts (you need just one nut daily to get an entire day's supply of this mineral), seafood, chicken, eggs, liver, red meat, and cereal grains. Because too much red meat is a risk factor for colorectal cancer, it's best to get your selenium mostly from plant sources.

Dosage: How Much Should You Take?

The recommended daily intake for selenium is 55 micrograms for men and woman over the age of nineteen. Normally, you get this amount from your diet. Multivitamin/mineral supplements usually contain 20 micrograms of selenium per tablet. The recommended dosage for antioxidant protection, however, is slightly higher: 100 to 200 micrograms a day.

Precautions

Never exceed a supplemental dosage of 200 micrograms daily, since higher doses can be toxic to the body.

OTHER SUPPLEMENTAL NUTRIENTS: VITAMIN E

Also garnering a lot of attention these days is vitamin E, an antioxidant that is present in the fat layers of cell membranes and works with selenium to protect cells from free radical damage.

Vitamin E and Colorectal Cancer

Claims that vitamin E protects against colorectal cancer or decreases the risk of polyps have yet to be substantiated, but the subject continues to be a fertile field of colorectal cancer research. What you may not know is that there are four major types of vitamin E called tocopherols, and each type may act differently on colon tissue. Researchers at the University of Utah evaluated these four types of vitamin E in a large group of men and women to see if the vitamin offered any protection. What emerged from this study was that alpha-tocopherol, the most active form, was slightly protective, but gamma-tocopherol—the most common form of vitamin E consumed by the people who were studied—slightly increased the risk of colorectal cancer.

Best Food Sources

Dietary sources of vitamin E include nuts, plant oils, leafy green vegetables, wheat germ, and fortified breakfast cereals. Some medical experts believe that it is difficult to obtain enough vitamin E from food, especially if you are following a low-fat diet, and for this reason supplementation is often recommended.

Dosage: How Much Should You Take?

There are a lot of unknowns right now with regard to vitamin E and colon cancer. Until we have more and better information on this vitamin, no one can convincingly make the case that supplemental vitamin E will protect healthy people from colorectal cancer. Vitamin E, however, is a very popular supplement that appears to offer protection against heart disease, and many doctors do recommend it for that reason.

Precautions

If you do take vitamin E, make sure you stop this supplement at least seven days before having any invasive procedure such as a colonoscopy. Like aspirin, vitamin E may increase your risk of bleeding.

ASPIRIN AND OTHER NONSTEROIDAL ANTI-INFLAMMATORY DRUGS (NSAIDS)

You have heard for years that aspirin—a true wonder drug and a member of a class of drugs known as nonsteroidal anti-inflammatory drugs, or NSAIDs—can keep heart attacks and stroke away. But did you know that it may work wonders against colorectal cancer, too?

That's right. One of the most exciting developments in colorectal cancer prevention involves aspirin and other NSAIDs.

For background, the spotlight on NSAIDs to fight cancer stems from the fact that the body has two versions of an enzyme termed cyclooxygenase, called COX-1 and COX-2 for short. Both enzymes help convert fatty acids into hormonelike chemicals called prostaglandins, involved in regulating numerous bodily processes. Prostaglandins arising from COX-1 reactions are required to maintain the lining of your stomach, promote the normal function of your kidneys, and slow blood clotting by interfering with platelets; prostaglandins arising from COX-2 reactions trigger inflammatory responses and the pain, swelling, or redness that so often accompanies inflammation. An excess of prostaglandins may be involved in cancerous tissue growth by disrupting the scheduled, orderly replacement of older cells with newer ones in the process called apoptosis. You see, even your cells are not supposed to live forever. The longer a cell is alive, the greater the chance that it will acquire mutations that may transform it into cancer. COX-2 activity, in particular, is involved in a process called angiogenesis, the formation of new blood vessels that nourish tumors, fostering their growth.

Aspirin and other familiar NSAIDs (namely ibuprofen, keto-profen, and naproxen sodium) interfere with the activity of COX-1 and COX-2 enzymes. The problem is that by inhibiting COX-1, traditional NSAIDs can lead to assorted side effects, including gastrointestinal bleeding and ulcer formation. Such troublesome side effects prompted the development of NSAIDs that inhibit only COX-2, and are less likely to cause gastrointestinal side effects. A new generation of NSAID was thus born—the COX-2 inhibitors, which include celecoxib (Celebrex), rofecoxib (Vioxx), and valde-coxib (Bextra).

NSAIDs and Colorectal Cancer

Here's a closer look at the science: Over the past twenty years, evidence from more than a hundred animal studies began demonstrating that aspirin and other NSAIDs could reduce the risk of colon and rectal cancers. More recently came large-population studies and clinical trials showing that aspirin and the newer NSAIDs had an equally protective effect in humans—lowering risk by up to 50 percent.

Two newly published studies, for example, found that taking an aspirin a day cuts the chances of developing precancerous polyps in people who have had colon cancer or are at a higher risk for it. In the first study, colon cancer survivors who took 325 milligrams of aspirin daily were much less likely to develop the type of polyp prone to turning into colon cancer. In the second, low-dose aspirin (81 milligrams a day) was protective in patients with a history of polyps. What's more, an American Cancer Society study of 662,000 adults found that people who took aspirin at least sixteen times a month were about half as likely to die of colon cancer as those who didn't use aspirin.

Since then, there have been many other studies pointing to a protective effect of aspirin—with one exception. The Physicians' Health Study found no association between aspirin and a decreased risk of colon cancer after five years of aspirin use. But most researchers feel that you need to take aspirin for decades—maybe even as long as twenty years—before your risk is reduced.

Another NSAID, sulindac (Clinoril), has been shown to reduce the number and size of polyps in patients with familial adenomatous polyps (FAP), the rare hereditary condition I discussed earlier in which the APC tumor suppressor gene is missing or defective. Even so, the benefit was short-lived, since follow-up research discovered that polyps returned and regrew three months after sulindac was discontinued.

Trials with the newer COX-2 inhibitors have been getting under way. One of the first looked into the benefits of giving Celebrex (400 milligrams a day) to patients with FAP. This study showed that Celebrex could reduce the number of polyps by nearly 30 percent. Celebrex has since been approved in the United States as part of the treatment of FAP.

This topic has particular interest to me since I am currently an investigator at Weill Cornell Medical College studying whether Celebrex can be used to help decrease the recurrence of polyps in patients who are found to have sporadic potentially precancerous adenomatous polyps. The concept here is that if COX-2 inhibition can decrease polyps in patients with FAP, and if COX-2 activation may be important for the formation of cancer, why not give a COX-2 inhibitor to people found to have random, sporadic adenomatous polyps? The results of this three-year trial are blinded (meaning the participants don't know whether they're taking a placebo or Celebrex) and will probably not be available until 2005.

The Anticancer Effect of NSAIDs

Exactly how do aspirin and other NSAIDs inhibit polyp and tumor growth in the first place? Many medical researchers believe that the anti-colon-cancer effect of these drugs most likely springs from their COX-2 inhibition. The COX-2 enzyme is elevated in colorectal polyps and tumors, suggesting that cancerous tissues need COX-2 to grow.

A 1999 study published in the *Journal of the American Medical Association* reported that colon tumors with the highest COX-2 levels were larger, more advanced, and more likely to spread to the lymph nodes. By contrast, COX-2 could not be detected in colon tissue from cancer-free patients.

NSAIDs stop the production of this enzyme and in doing so may prevent colorectal cancer from developing in the first place. (Worth mentioning here: acetaminophen, better known as Tylenol, is a drug often given as an NSAID substitute. It does not, however, demonstrate any protection against colorectal cancer.)

The results of research into colorectal cancer and aspirin, NSAIDs, and specific COX-2 inhibitors are very promising and have spurred much continued study. I feel that the prospect of using COX-2 inhibitors to prevent and treat colon cancer is exciting. But we are just scratching the surface and there is so much we still do not know.

Caution should be exercised here, since the right amount of COX-1 and COX-2 enzymes may be critical for keeping your body in balance. If you were to inhibit all COX activity—which can happen with long-term use of NSAIDs—you might jeopardize the health of your organs and overall functioning. Nor are we certain yet whether these drugs prevent the development of colorectal cancer in healthy people, or just in people with a genetic predisposition.

Should You Take NSAIDs?

I hesitate to give a blanket recommendation for taking aspirin or other NSAIDs solely to prevent colorectal cancer—unless you have been diagnosed as having FAP or you are considered by your doctor to be at high risk for developing polyps or colorectal cancer. If you are prescribed aspirin for protection from a heart attack or stroke, certainly you gain the "fringe benefit" of colon cancer protection. In the same vein, if you are prescribed an NSAID or COX-2 inhibitor for arthritis, you may get an added anticancer benefit.

Precautions

Why don't we all just take these wonder drugs to help reduce our risk for colorectal cancer? The answer is simple: As wondrous as they are, there are some very serious complications that can occur with the use of these drugs. Life-threatening ulceration and gastrointestinal bleeding can occur suddenly and painlessly while taking aspirin and other NSAIDs. Although COX-2 inhibitors are thought to be safer for the gastrointestinal tract, they may still cause problems. No one knows this better than a gastroenterologist like myself. If someone develops severe bleeding on any of these drugs, I am the one who is called in the middle of the night to do an emergency endoscopy (a procedure that looks directly into the stomach and intestine) to locate the source of bleeding and cauterize any affected blood vessels.

Depending on what your general state of health is or what (if any) medications you're taking, there are some additional guidelines you should follow to prevent any complications from using aspirin and NSAIDs:

- If you are allergic to aspirin or NSAIDs, or suffer from ulcers, gastritis, or any inflammatory stomach or gastrointestinal disorders, avoid medications containing NSAIDs—they can trigger potentially dangerous complications.
- If you are preparing for surgery or another procedure (including a colonoscopy), do not take aspirin or NSAIDs for at least one week before, because they can increase bleeding during your operation or procedure. Your physician may recommend an alternative medicine if you require one.
- Do not mix aspirin with other drugs. These include other NSAIDs, anticoagulants, corticosteroids, heparin, and gout medication.
- If you bruise or bleed easily, or experience burning in your stomach, abdominal pain, or black tarry stools, stop taking the aspirin or NSAID, and notify your doctor immediately or go to the nearest emergency room.

THE NEWS ON NATURAL NSAIDS

Sitting in your spice rack may be a seasoning that is a powerful medicinal herb: turmeric, one of the major spices in curry powder and one of the best-studied of the anti-inflammatory herbs. Turmeric contains curcumin, a yellow pigment that is the active ingredient in this herb. Widely used medicinally in Asian countries such as India and Pakistan, curcumin may be partially responsible for the lower rate of colon and rectal cancers in these regions of the world. In cells cultured in lab dishes as well as in animal studies, curcumin has been shown to inhibit COX-2, arrest cancer cells in various stages of formation, and act as an antioxidant. Other research, however, indicates that curcumin may have pro-oxidant effects, meaning that it promotes disease-causing free radicals.

Other natural agents that may possibly inhibit COX-2 include red ginseng, rosemary, and catechins in green tea. These herbs are in the early stages of investigation. Until long-term human trials are conducted, it is too early to tell whether these herbs will pan out as natural agents for preventing colorectal cancer.

I am open to herbal treatments as long as I see solid proof of their effectiveness—in other words, sound scientific evidence from human clinical trials. I always advise patients to approach any herbal remedy with caution. Herbs such as curcumin are agents to watch; however, it is premature to start recommending them to ward off colorectal cancer.

HORMONE REPLACEMENT THERAPY (HRT)

To my women readers: Just when you thought the news about hormone replacement therapy was all bad, now comes the news that it decreases the risk of colorectal cancer—by maybe 20 to 30 percent, or even more.

HRT, which involves the use of estrogen with or without the hormone progestin, has been widely used to treat symptoms of menopause and prevent chronic illnesses such as heart disease and osteoporosis. But in 2001, alarms sounded when the National Institutes of Health (NIH) halted part of its Women's Health Initiative, a massive research trial of HRT, citing that the increased risk of heart attack, stroke, and breast cancer outweighed the benefits of bone protection and lower colorectal cancer rates.

Where colorectal cancer is concerned, the protective benefits seem to stem from estrogen. But exactly how estrogen helps avert colorectal cancer has stumped scientists. From a cellular perspective, it may halt the inactivation of tumor suppressor genes, prevent inadequate DNA repair, or induce apoptosis (programmed cell death). In addition, estrogen may decrease levels of bile acids and slow down the production of insulin-like growth factor, a chemical researchers believe might promote colon cancer. Estrogen may even interfere with COX-2 activity.

So women, with their higher estrogen levels compared to men, must have a lower rate of colorectal cancer, right? *Wrong!* The fact is that men and women have similar rates of colorectal cancer. I am actually at a loss to give a good explanation for this discrepancy. There may be some gender difference in rates of polyp formation and the rate of malignant transformation of polyps, but this is all speculation at the current time.

So where does this leave you, especially if you are trying to relieve menopausal symptoms or protect yourself from osteoporosis? The whole issue of whether women should be on any form of HRT is a thorny one. In some cases, there may be valid medical reasons to support a hormonal strategy for combating colorectal cancer, particularly in cases where there is a strong family history. You must keep in mind that when you take hormones, there's always a trade-off in terms of potentially harmful side effects. But if you're a woman whose family history places you at high risk for colorectal cancer, the idea of HRT can be addressed with your physician, especially if there is another reason that you might benefit from HRT.

What I think is absolutely critical is that your doctor discuss with you the increasing number of other options for preventing colorectal cancer without resorting to HRT and the risks it potentially raises. These strategies include regular screenings, lifestyle adjustments, diet, and the many measures I've discussed with you in this chapter. The bottom line is that you need to weigh the pros and cons of any intervention with great care, and always in consultation with your physician.

Table 6-1

Dr. Pochapin's Supplementation and Chemoprevention Guide

Supplement	Natural Sources	Dosage
Folic Acid	Dark green leafy vegetables (spinach, kale, romaine lettuce), asparagus, broccoli, brussels sprouts, lima beans, peas, sweet potatoes, cantaloupe, oranges, oatmeal, wheat germ, fortified grains and cereals, wild rice, liver.	Take 400 micrograms daily as part of a multivitamin supplement.
Calcium	Dairy products, spinach, collard greens, broccoli, tofu, almonds.	Take 1,000 milligrams a day if you're between 19 and 50; and 1,200 milligrams a day if you're older than 50. Do not exceed 1,500 milligrams a day (diet and supplement combined). You should definitely take supplemental calcium if you have osteoporosis. Avoid calcium if you have a history of kidney stones. I do not recommend calcium supplementation for men due to the possible association with prostate cancer.
Vitamin D	Sun exposure, fatty saltwater fish (tuna, halibut, mackerel, herring, sardines), fortified milk, enriched cereals, maitake and shiitake mushrooms.	Take 200 IUs daily if you are 19 to 50; 400 IUs daily if you are 51 to 70; and 600 IUs daily if you are older than 70. Try to get 15 minutes of sunlight each day, if possible.
Selenium	Brazil nuts, seafood, chicken, eggs, liver, red meat, cereals.	Take up to 50 to 100 micrograms daily.
Vitamin E	Nuts, plant oils, leafy green vegetables, wheat germ, fortified cereals.	Take 200 to 400 IUs daily.
NSAIDs (including aspirin)	Turmeric. (Studies are being conducted on red ginseng, rosemary, and green tea.)	Consider taking an NSAID if you have a family history of colon cancer. Do not take these drugs unless you discuss this course of action with your physician. These drugs can cause serious adverse effects such as bleeding ulcers.
Hormone replacement therapy (HRT)	None.	Discuss your personal situation, such as family history of colon cancer, with your physician, but look to other supplemental approaches as a better first line of defense.

MY PARTING MESSAGE ON SUPPLEMENTATION AND CHEMOPREVENTION

What I am advocating is a sensible, straightforward approach to supplementation and chemoprevention. I believe that nutrients such as folic acid, calcium, and vitamin D, if taken daily as a part of a preventive plan that includes exercise and proper diet, have value in helping to prevent colorectal cancer or its recurrence. Keep in mind that the agents I've discussed here may modify your risk of developing colorectal cancer, but they certainly have not been proven to prevent it, cure it, or keep it from coming back. While these agents are certainly a logical "insurance policy" they are not a guarantee or magic bullet. You can't take folic acid, calcium, aspirin, or anything else and believe you're protected. Most importantly, supplementation and chemoprevention is not a substitute or excuse to avoid seeing your doctor or getting screened.

Part III

HOPE FOR A BETTER TOMORROW: FROM DIAGNOSIS TO TREATMENT

Chapter 7

Getting a Diagnosis:
Understanding Pathology and Staging

The actual diagnosis of colorectal cancer requires a bit of medical detective work, depending on whether or not your doctor finds anything during your colonoscopy or other screening test. Maybe you were sent home with a clean bill of colon health. Maybe your doctor removed one or two polyps. Maybe your doctor found a bigger growth that will have to be removed surgically.

Whatever the situation, any tissue that is removed must be studied microscopically, for the presence of precancerous or cancerous cells, to determine whether a growth is benign or malignant, or to learn how far a tumor has spread.

What we will look at in this chapter is how colorectal cancer is diagnosed: what a pathologist looks for, how to understand the pathology report you receive from the pathologist, and how your doctor "stages" colorectal cancer. Staging describes how far a newly discovered cancer has spread. There are emotional issues attached to a diagnosis of colorectal cancer as well. How to cope with a diagnosis of cancer is a subject I will take up in chapter 8.

DIAGNOSING COLORECTAL CANCER: THE ROLE OF THE PATHOLOGIST

A pathologist is a medical doctor who specializes in the evaluation of tissue in order to diagnose disease. Although you will never meet your pathologist, he or she is an important part of the diagnosis and treatment team for colorectal cancer.

If your doctor removed a polyp during your examination, the entire polyp is sent to the pathologist. The pathologist studies the polyp tissue under a microscope, evaluating many of its characteristics and detailing these features in a written pathology report. This report, often referred to as the path report, is usually available within a week of having your colonoscopy or flexible sigmoidoscopy.

Ask your doctor if you can see your path report so that you can ask questions about the results. It is your right to have access to your test results, and most doctors will be more than happy to give you a copy for your records. The reports are an excellent means of documenting when the procedure was performed and what was found. I think one reason people don't ask for these reports is that they're afraid that they won't comprehend all the medical lingo. I intend to clear that up by showing you how to read your pathology reports and better understand your diagnosis. It's really not as perplexing as you might think.

UNDERSTANDING YOUR ENDOSCOPIC PATH REPORT

On your endoscopic path report, the pathologist will describe a polyp according to the following characteristics.

Polyp Site

This part of the report will note the location from which the polyp was removed—information supplied by your doctor when he or she removed the polyp. Occasionally, the exact location is not known, and the physician may designate it by measuring the number of centimeters from the rectum to the general area from which the polyp was taken.

Polyp Size

The polyp is measured as a part of the pathology evaluation. The larger the polyp, the greater the likelihood that it may be cancerous. The polyp size on a path report is often smaller than that described by the doctor who removed it due to the preservative and lack of blood supply. Polyps measuring one centimeter or more in diameter may be a cause for concern. In the world of a polyp, size does matter.

Polyp Configuration

This part of the report describes the general shape of the polyp—another factor that influences its odds of being cancerous. Specifically, the pathologist will note whether the polyp is sessile (flat) or pedunculated (protruded), with or without a stalk. If there is a stalk, the stalk may be measured. Again, this is very important information. Pedunculated polyps are less suspicious than sessile polyps.

Histologic Type—No Cancer Present

The pathologist studies the polyp under a microscope to see the type of cells present. If no cancer is seen, the polyp is classified in one of three ways: hyperplastic, inflammatory, or adenomatous.

   • **Hyperplastic polyps** are usually very small (about the size of a pea), completely benign, and, like a bump on your skin, simply an overgrowth of normal tissue.

   • **Inflammatory polyps** are also small and benign. They are made up of a collection of inflamed cells and may be associated with inflammatory bowel disease (ulcerative colitis or Crohn's disease).

   • **Adenomatous polyps** are a different story altogether, since they have the potential to turn into cancer—which is why this type of polyp is best described as "potentially precancerous." Adenomatous polyps are the most common type of polyp, found in roughly 10 to 25 percent of people by age fifty. If your doctor happened to remove a polyp found by the pathologist to be adenomatous, that's very good news. Why good news? Well, by getting rid of that adenomatous polyp, the possibility of it developing into colorectal cancer has been halted. In other words, cancer may have been prevented!

To sum up, if the polyp that was removed turns out to be hyperplastic, inflammatory, or adenomatous, you're in the clear. And that is very good news indeed.

Histologic Type—Precancerous or Cancer Cells Present

If the polyp contains precancerous or cancerous cells, the report will describe these cells in one of three ways:

• **Adenocarcinoma.** This describes cancer cells that arise from the normal cells lining the colon or rectum. Adenocarcinoma is the most common type of colon and rectal cancers observed.

• **Carcinoma in situ.** These are cells that show very early cancerous changes on the surface only. If treated early, they are less likely to spread.

• **Dysplasia.** This term describes precancerous changes seen in abnormal cells. Cells that show signs of dysplasia are believed to be on their way to turning cancerous.

Histologic Dysplasia Grade

Pathologists and physicians mention "histologic grade" only if dysplasia is present. The grade of a polyp describes the degree or severity of dysplasia in the cells. *Low-grade dysplasia* indicates that the precancerous cells are less aggressive. *High-grade dysplasia,* on the other hand, means that the precancerous cells are growing fast and are on the verge of turning cancerous.

Degree of Differentiation

In cancer, *differentiation* describes how well developed cancer cells are. A *well or moderately differentiated adenocarcinoma* refers to cancer cells that resemble normal cells and tend to grow and spread at a lower rate than a poorly differentiated adenocarcinoma. Poorly differentiated cells lack the structure and function of normal cells and tend to grow more uncontrollably.

Extent of Invasion

This term is usually reserved for describing dysplasia or carcinoma within a polyp that has been removed during a colonoscopy or surgery. In the report, the pathologist describes the depth of invasion of dysplasia or carcinoma from within the polyp. Often, dysplasia and carcinoma travel down the polyp into its stalk and underlying colon lining.

If the cancer has invaded the wall of your colon or rectum, you will need to have surgical resection of that piece of bowel and surrounding lymph nodes. An additional pathological examination will be performed on the surgical specimens to determine the stage (see below).

Margins

If cancerous cells are present, the pathologist microscopically checks the margins of the polyps to determine whether these cells have migrated to the edges of or beyond the polyp itself.

THE SURGICAL PATH REPORT

If your doctor found a tumor in your colon or rectum, you'll undergo surgery to remove the growth, and possibly a section of your colon or rectum and surrounding lymph nodes. The pathologist will perform a microscope evaluation of those tissues as well. I will talk in more detail about surgery in chapter 9, but for the purposes of our discussion here, I want to focus on what a pathologist looks for in a surgical specimen and how it is reported.

The surgical path report describes the tumor, sections of your colon, lymph nodes, and other tissue samples that were removed during surgery.

Type and Size of Sample Removed for Biopsy

This part of the report will note the location from which the tumor was removed, and whether any tissue besides the tumor was taken out. The pathologist will also measure the size of the tumor.

Tumor Configuration

Not all tumors look alike. Some are ulcerated because they have deep ulcer craters on the surface. Other tumors are described according to their growth pattern. For example, bulky tumors are often termed fungating.

Histologic Type

It's not so much a tumor's size or shape that determines how quickly it will grow, but rather its underlying cellular biology. This part of the report notes the type of cancer cells present. As with malignant polyps, tumor cells are described as adenocarcinoma. Carcinoma in situ and/or dysplasia may also be described. Other aspects of the tumor will be reported, too. For instance, if the tumor secretes a lot of mucus or has the appearance of signet cells, this may indicate a more aggressive tumor. (Cells with a rim and a thickened interior are known as signet cells because they resemble a signet ring.)

Histologic Grade

This part of the report describes differentiation in terms of degree: *poorly, moderately,* or *well differentiated.* Poorly differentiated cells are the most aggressive of the three types; moderately differentiated cells are less aggressive; and well-differentiated cells are the least aggressive and suggest the best prognosis of the three.

Presence or Absence of Lymphatic Vessel Invasion

This condition means that the cancer cells have invaded the walls of the lymphatic vessels and have the potential to travel to your lymph nodes.

Presence or Absence of Blood Vessel Invasion

This information tells you and your doctor whether the cancer cells have invaded the walls of the small blood vessels that surround the tumor. If they have, this means that there is a greater potential for cancer cells to reach the bloodstream and migrate to other organs. If your doctor suspects that cancer has spread to other parts of your body, he or she will order other diagnostic tests, such as a computerized tomography (CT) scan, magnetic resonance imaging (MRI), ultrasound, or a positron emission tomography (PET) scan to confirm these suspicions. The spread of cancer to another part of the body is termed *metastasis*.

Margins

These are the edges of the tissue sample removed, and they are analyzed for evidence of cancer cells. If the cancer was able to be completely excised, the margins should be free of cancer cells.

Extent of Tumor Invasion

This very important part of the report describes how far a tumor has penetrated the layers of the colon or rectal wall. What's more, it reflects your prognosis and whether you may need chemotherapy. A tumor that is confined to the inner layer has a better prognosis and is more curable than one that has infiltrated through all the layers of the colon or rectum. In addition, chemotherapy may not be required for a cancer that has not penetrated through the colon wall. The deeper the tumor penetrates the colon or rectum, the greater the chance it has of spreading to the lymph nodes and metastisizing to other sites in the body.

Status of Lymph Nodes

The report will state whether the lymph nodes are positive or negative. *Negative* means that no cancer cells have been found in your lymph nodes; *positive* means that lymph nodes contain cancer cells. The report will also indicate the location and number of the lymph nodes and how many were found to have cancer cells.

Once the cancer has been removed by surgery, analyzed microscopically, and described by the pathologist in the surgical path report, this information will be put together with other tests so that your doctor can categorize your cancer according to a stage. Staging is vital because it helps determine the type of treatment you will have, your chances of a cure, and your long-term prognosis or outcome.

THE STAGES OF COLORECTAL CANCER

Staging assigns a letter and number code to the tumor in order to tell your doctor how involved your cancer may be in your colon, rectum, and surrounding structures. Put another way, staging identifies the extent of the tumor's infiltration into healthy tissue and lymph nodes at the time of diagnosis. Your treatment and your prognosis, to a certain extent, both depend on the stage of your cancer. With early-stage cancer, for example, surgery may be the only treatment required, whereas in more advanced stages chemotherapy or radiation may be needed. Your doctor should thoroughly explain the stage to you so that you can be informed and involved in your own treatment decisions when it comes time to make them. Coupled with the diagnosis made from the pathology reports will be the results of other medical tests your doctor has ordered. These are tests that I will summarize for you in the next chapter.

In the staging of colon and rectal cancer, more than one system is used. The most widely used is the tumor node metastasis (TNM) system, which describes stages using Roman numerals I through IV. Another is the Dukes-Kirklin system, an older system that uses the letters A through D. Both systems give the same basic information: the extent of the spread of cancer in relation to the walls of the colon or rectum, nearby organs, and other organs farther away. When I teach fellows—doctors training to be gastroenterologists—at the Weill Medical College of Cornell University, I use the TNM classification, but the Dukes-Kirklin system is often still referred to by physicians, so you should be familiar with both.

With the TNM system, the letter designations *T, N,* and *M* are used as a code to describe the depth of the tumor's invasion into surrounding tissue (T designation), whether it has spread to lymph node or nodes (N designation); and the extent of the cancer's metastatic spread to other organs (M designation). Table 7-1 describes the T, N, and M categories in greater detail.

Table 7-1

How to Understand the T, N, and M Categories

T Categories for Colorectal Cancer

T_x	The tumor's extent cannot be described because of incomplete information.
T_0	No evidence of a primary (original) tumor.
T_{is}	The cancer is in its earliest stage; it has not grown beyond the mucosa (inner layer) of the colon or rectum. The *is* stands for "in situ."
T_1	The cancer has grown through the mucosa and extends into the submucosa.
T_2	The cancer has grown through the submucosa and extends into the muscle layer but does not penetrate through it.
T_3	The cancer has grown completely through the muscle layer. It has not spread to any nearby organs or tissues.
T_4	The cancer has spread completely through the wall of the colon or rectum and into nearby organs or tissues.

N Categories for Colorectal Cancer

N_x	No description of lymph node involvement because of incomplete information.
N_0	No lymph node involvement.
N_1	Cancer cells have been detected in 1 to 3 nearby lymph nodes.
N_2	Cancer cells have been detected in 4 or more nearly lymph nodes.
N_3	Cancer cells have been detected in lymph nodes along a major blood vessel, and/or have spread to the lymph node at the top of the blood vessel.

M Categories for Colorectal Cancer

M_x	No description of distant spread is possible because of incomplete information.
M_0	The cancer has not spread to distant sites.
M_1	The cancer has spread to distant sites.

Once your T, N, and M categories have been determined, this information is put together in a process called stage grouping, expressed in Roman numerals from stage 0 (the least advanced stage) to stage IV (the most advanced stage). When written out, the letters *T, N,* and *M* are followed by their respective number designation. So, for example, a T designation of category 3 is a T_3.

Specifically, here's how the TNM categories, along with their Dukes-Kirklin equivalent, are grouped together in stages:

Stage 0

• $T_{is}N_0M_0$: Your cancer is in its earliest stage. It has not progressed beyond the inner layer (mucosa) of the colon or rectum. This stage is also called carcinoma in situ; the *is* stands for "in situ," meaning "in its usual place."

Stage I

• $T_1N_0M_0$ = Dukes-Kirklin A: The cancer has spread beyond the mucosa into the next layer, called the submucosa, of the colon or rectum, but it has not yet spread outside the colon wall into the nearby lymph nodes (N_0) or organs (M_0).

• $T_2N_0M_0$ = Dukes-Kirklin B1: The cancer has grown into the next layer, called the muscularis propria (the muscle layer of the colon) but it has not spread to nearby lymph nodes or metastasized to other organs.

Stages 0 and I have the best prognosis, or predicted outcome. Statistically, about 96 percent of people in this stage are doing fine five years after initial surgical resection. Chemotherapy is usually not required for these early stage I cancers.

Stage II

• $T_3N_0M_0$ or $T_4N_0M_0$ = Dukes-Kirklin B2: In this stage, the cancer has spread through the muscularis of the colon or rectum, but has not yet spread to any lymph nodes. If T_4, the tumor may have invaded neighboring organs or structures, however. Stage II has a fairly good prognosis. About 87 percent of patients diagnosed in stage II will live at least five years after their initial treatment.

Stage III

- $T_xN_1M_0$ = **Dukes-Kirklin C:** This is a more advanced stage of colon or rectal cancer. The cancer is present in one to three lymph nodes near the colon or rectum (N_1), but there is no evidence that it has migrated to other organs (M_0). The designation T_x is another way of saying that the cancer can be "any T," meaning that the tumor's penetration does not affect the stage. Some staging reports may indicate N_2 or N_3; this means the cancer has spread to nearby lymph nodes. In this stage, about 55 percent of patients are alive five years after their initial treatment.

Stage IV

- $T_xN_xM_1$ = **Dukes-Kirklin D.** The cancer can be any T, any N, but it has metastasized to distant tissues and organs. The most common site for metastasis is the liver, although cancer can spread to the peritoneum (the membrane enveloping the abdomen), lung, brain, or ovary. Stage IV has a poor prognosis. About 5 percent of patients with stage IV cancer are alive five years after their initial treatment.

Let me emphasize here, though, that these stage-by-stage survival rates are only prognostic predictors, based on the law of averages. They do not reflect the new discoveries and treatments that you will read about in this book. Miracles can and do happen, so do not let the news that you have a late-stage cancer destroy your hope. Hope is your greatest ally, and do not let any doctor or statistic take that away from you!

Chapter 8

Dealing with Your Diagnosis and Choosing Dr. Right

Should you find out for sure that you have colorectal cancer, the days and weeks after your diagnosis and preceding your treatment can be a time of anxiety and uncertainty. But these emotions are not insurmountable. Learning to cope emotionally with your diagnosis, selecting the right doctor and treatment facility, and becoming familiar with your treatment options can help you regain a sense of control over your life and help you focus on beating this disease.

COPING WITH YOUR DIAGNOSIS

If one of my patients is diagnosed with cancer, I always try to report these results in person, not over the telephone but right in my office. If your pathology results show cancer a caring physician will invite you in for a personal, face-to-face discussion, so you can ask questions and get answers. This is important because the doctor—patient partnership depends on both sides being open and honest.

Now, if life does deal you a diagnosis of colorectal cancer, you'll feel a range of emotions, depending on your particular case. You may feel relieved, thankful, and reassured if your doctor tells you that your cancer has not spread, and that with surgery, you have a great chance of being cured. On the other hand, if your cancer is more advanced, you may feel devastated, in shock, depressed, fearful, unable to comprehend anything other than the fact that you have colorectal cancer. Whatever emotions you feel, they are normal and they are understandable.

When working with my own patients, I have a heart-to-heart discussion with them about ways to make it through this emotional time in their lives. The advice I give to them, I hope will also help you.

Focus on the Positive

Maybe your cancer was caught early, which means that it is in its most curable stage. Or maybe your cancer is in an advanced stage—but now that you know its stage, the most appropriate treatment can be mapped out so that you will be on the path to a cure. Remember, there is plenty of colorectal cancer that can be cured, and every day is another day of hope that a new treatment might be available. Concentrate on these and other positives in your life. Doing so lifts your spirit and amplifies your immune response so that you are better able to heal and to respond to treatment.

What's more, developing a positive, constructive frame of mind gives you a sense of control that will keep stress chemicals from reaching damaging levels while you are dealing with your diagnosis and undergoing subsequent treatment. By contrast, a sense of helplessness and a giving-up reaction can cause a severe and disabling clinical depression and a weakening of your immune system. Of course, you will certainly have bad days with times of sadness or fear. Don't expect to be positive all the time—it is just not realistic. Rather, focus on taking care of yourself and visualize getting well.

Trust me, hope can grow even in the midst of something as ominous as cancer. I believe that your own inner strength, nourished by the love and support of others, can conquer anything. I personally have witnessed some of the most beautiful expressions of human behavior in the setting of the most devastating of cancers. People who have a powerful belief in themselves, a strong desire to live, and a reluctance to give up hope often outlive their predicted life expectancies, or survive the cancer altogether. Draw from your own reservoir of emotional and spiritual strength and embrace the love of family and friends. You will find that the same fighting spirit can be yours. You can do it! So many others have.

Talk It Out

Pour your heart out to your significant other, a family member, or an understanding and sympathetic friend. Most of us think we are alone and unique in our trials and suffering, but these feelings only impede our ability to heal. Having frank and confiding relationships, even with just one or two people, will release your anxieties and fears, so tell a couple of trusted people in your life how you feel. Getting your feelings out in the open is a positive emotional move—and one that will make it easier to cope.

Stay Connected with Those Going Through the Same Ordeal

Find a support group where you can talk to other people who have had colorectal cancer. Organizations that can provide this contact are listed in "Resources," at the end of this book. This can help alleviate the feelings of despair and hopelessness that so frequently accompany a diagnosis of cancer. Getting involved in a support group can sustain you not only as you deal with your diagnosis but also throughout your treatment and beyond.

These moments of connection with other people can blossom forth to give you a feeling of strength, control, and hope. You may like to think that you can get through this on your own, but no one can. Trust me on this one. You *need* other people to help you through this. Among these people should be your doctor and your medical team.

YOUR DOCTOR AND YOUR MEDICAL TEAM

Faced with a serious diagnosis such as colorectal cancer and the treatment it requires, you will need to be under the care of a great doctor and a great medical team. At this point, you probably have a gastroenterologist who discovered your cancer during a colonoscopy. If your gastroenterologist removed a polyp during a colonoscopy, and this is all the care you required, you will not need further treatment. Nor will you need the services of any other medical specialists. You will need, however, to undergo follow-up colonoscopies in the future to check for new polyps.

If, however, you require surgery and/or chemotherapy or radiation, then your gastroenterologist should refer you to a surgeon, an oncologist (cancer specialist), or both. In fact, you'll be seeing a team comprising several different doctors and other medical professionals. These will include an oncologist, your gastroenterologist, a radiologist, a surgeon, and a pathologist.

Although each physician plays a different role in your care and looks at cancer from a unique perspective, one doctor should be in charge of coordinating your entire treatment plan. Like a well-trained football team, your medical team may have the very best players, but unless it has a quarterback—a doctor who orchestrates the plays—the entire medical experience lacks coordination, and this can create undue stress for you. So as you begin treatment, find out which doctor will be your quarterback. Initially, this will probably be your gastroenterologist. Quarterbacking may shift among the different specialists involved, however. For example, the surgeon will oversee your care until your recovery from surgery is complete. If your cancer was invasive and requires chemotherapy or radiation, an oncologist may become the quarterback of your treatment team following your surgery. Regardless of who is in charge, you'll want to make sure you have the very best.

FINDING A DOCTOR

Some doctors are brilliant and masters at the technical side of medicine. Others may have a soothing, warm bedside manner and a presence that generates confidence and comfort. What you want in your doctor is a combination of these qualities—a person who is competent, compassionate, and great at communication.

How do you find such a doctor?

Well, it takes a bit of luck, some research, and word of mouth. If you are a member of a health insurance plan, your choice may be limited to those doctors who participate in your plan. Even so, you can still evaluate the doctors in your plan according to a checklist.

Referrals and Recommendations

As I mentioned earlier, your gastroenterologist or your primary care physician will most likely refer you to a surgeon who specializes in colon and rectal surgery. Most people pick the first surgeon who is recommended to them and go to the hospital where he or she happens to be affiliated. That's fine for simple operations and procedures such as colonoscopies, but colorectal surgery is more complicated and requires specialized training and technique. If you're the one hopping on the operating table, you want to make sure you do your homework and choose the very best surgeon you can find.

Board-Certified

If your doctor recommends a surgeon or oncologist, check the physician's credentials to ascertain whether he or she is board-certified, since board certification indicates that physicians are well qualified in their fields of medicine and stay current in their specialties. You'll want to find a surgeon who is board-certified in colon and rectal surgery by the American Board of Colon and Rectal Surgery. In addition to being proficient in the field of general surgery, a board-certified colon and rectal surgeon has acquired special skills and knowledge in the medical and surgical management of diseases of the colon, rectum, and other parts of the intestinal tract. Another option is to select a surgeon who is board-certified in surgical oncology by the American Board of Surgery. These surgeons have special training in several types of surgical procedures, including biopsy, tumor staging, and tumor resection (removal).

Oncologists are medical physicians who specialize in the treatment of cancer. There are several types of board certification for oncologists. Important in the medical treatment for colorectal cancer is finding an oncologist who is board-certified by the American

Board of Internal Medicine in medical oncology. The American Board of Radiology examines and board-certifies radiation oncologists, who specialize in the radiation therapy for cancer.

These medical organizations have Web sites where you can locate a board-certified surgeon or oncologist in your community, and these are listed in "Resources." Another good source is the American Board of Medical Specialties (ABMS). It publishes a list of board-certified physicians, with doctors' names along with their specialty and their educational background. The ABMS also has a Web site that can be used to verify a physician's board certification. This Web site in listed in "Resources" as well.

During your search for a doctor, you may also run across doctors who are board-eligible. This usually means they are younger and have had the required education and training, but have not yet completed the board examination. I would only recommend board-eligible doctors if they practice in a group with more senior physicians who are board-certified.

Volume

For surgery in particular, look for a board-certified surgeon who does colorectal surgery often. Doctors who frequently perform certain surgeries or procedures can operate with experience and confidence. There are a couple of ways you can track this down. One is to contact your local medical society to see if it keeps a record of such information. If the medical society doesn't have it, simply ask the surgeon you're considering how many times he or she performs the procedure each year.

Advice from Friends and Relatives

Talk to any friends and relatives who have been treated for colorectal cancer to find out which doctors they recommend. Listening to their advice is a good idea, but treat it with caution. If someone you know was thorough in finding a physician, then you can be more confident about his or her choice.

Hospital Affiliations

Check out the hospitals in your area. Good doctors are usually affiliated with good hospitals. (See the next section for information on how to select a hospital or treatment facility.) You can find out this information by calling the physician's office, then verifying it with the hospital.

The best doctors also tend to be affiliated with the large academic teaching institutions, although these hospitals may be far from your home. In this case, you may want to travel to get an opinion at one of these institutions but have your care given by more local doctors.

You may have already chosen a hospital for your treatment. If so, make sure the doctor you're considering can use the hospital you've selected.

First Impressions

The first meeting with a prospective surgeon or oncologist will give you enough facts and firsthand information to help you decide if you want to become this doctor's patient. For, example, when you see the doctor, is he or she friendly and responsive, or preoccupied? Does the doctor explain things clearly and encourage you to ask questions? Does the doctor listen to you, treat you with respect, and show an interest in your emotional health? The better physicians can comfort and communicate with their patients. They are interested in treating the whole person, not just the colon or rectum. If these qualities aren't there, start shopping around for another doctor.

SELECTING A HOSPITAL OR CANCER TREATMENT CENTER

Selecting an excellent treatment facility is as important as selecting a great doctor. It is vital to be familiar with the hospitals or cancer treatment centers (which are often affiliated with hospitals) in your community, including the ones that are covered by your insurance plan. Here's a checklist of what to look for:

• **Treatment program:** Does the facility have a treatment program for colorectal cancer? This means that qualified gastroenterologists, surgeons, medical oncologists, and other health care professionals are on staff to coordinate your treatment plan and follow-up care.

• **Accreditation:** Find out whether the hospital is accredited by the Joint Commission on Accreditation of Healthcare Organizations (JCAHO), meaning that it has met the standards for quality care. You can determine this by calling the hospital directly, or by visiting the JCAHO Web site, listed in "Resources."

Another accrediting body is the American College of Surgeons (ACOS). The ACOS accredits cancer programs at hospitals and other treatment facilities. To date, more than fourteen hundred programs in the United States have been accredited by ACOS. The organization's Web site maintains a searchable database of these programs. (See "Resources" for ACOS's Web site and other important contact information.)

• **Volume:** How often does the hospital perform the particular procedure or operation you need? Again, I'm talking about volume. Plenty of research shows that hospitals that perform a high volume of certain procedures are more competent, with a better success rate, than hospitals that do the procedure infrequently. To find out, ask your surgeon how often the procedure is performed at the hospital.

Please do not be timid about asking hospitals for information, either. What your doctor or other health care professionals may not tell you up front is that as a patient, you have rights. The American Hospital Association established in 1973 a Patient's Bill of Rights, and updated it in 1992. All accredited hospitals must abide by this bill, which covers twelve rights, including your right to quality of care, privacy, and information regarding diagnosis, treatment, and prognosis. Under the Patient's Bill of Rights, you also have the right to refuse a recommended treatment and plan of care, and you have the right to be transferred to another hospital if you request it.

If it is convenient and feasible for you, you may want to select one of the best hospitals as listed in the *U.S. News and World Report* Web site at www.usnews.com, or one of the National Cancer Institute's (NCI) fifty medical centers for your treatment. These facilities provide state-of-the-art diagnosis and treatment, conduct research in cancer, and investigate new methods of treatment.

You can obtain information about referral procedures, treatment, costs, and services by logging on to the NCI's Web site, which features a list of individual cancer centers, with addresses and telephone numbers. (The NCI Web site is listed in "Resources.")

Regarding insurance: You or someone working on your behalf should find out if your insurance company will cover everything you need for your care. All scheduled appointments, procedures, and hospitalizations should be cleared with your insurance company *before* you start any treatment.

THE TEAM APPROACH: MAXIMIZE YOUR CHANCES OF GETTING THE BEST CARE

Your "quarterback" doctor will organize and coordinate a team of professionals to treat and care for you—before you begin treatment, while you are hospitalized, and during the period required for recovery and follow-up care. This team includes not only you and your family, but also a variety of other individuals trained to deal with specific aspects of colorectal cancer. In addition to your gastroenterologist, surgeon, and oncologist, this team generally consists of the following.

Radiologist

Unlike other medical doctors, the radiologist diagnoses disease and monitors the effect of treatment by obtaining and interpreting medical images from CT scans, MRIs, ultrasound, and other types of scans. The radiologist takes the findings of medical images, correlates them with other exams and tests, recommends further tests, and consults with your doctor in order to provide the most appropriate care. In essence, a radiologist serves as your doctor's doctor by providing assistance through the interpreting of medical imaging. Although you may never see your radiologist, he or she plays a vital role in your diagnosis, treatment, and follow-up care.

Radiation Oncologist

One special type of physician you may see if you have rectal cancer is a radiation oncologist. Radiation oncologists are subspecialists who use radiation therapy to treat cancer.

Nurses

Truly the angels of medicine, nurses are responsible for implementing the plan of care ordered by your doctor. In the setting of hospitalized care, a good nurse can make all the difference in the world! Nurses administer your medications, assess your symptoms, monitor your intravenous (IV) lines, check your vital signs, supervise dressing changes, and take care of your personal hygiene, among many other important duties. Your nurses will also assess your pain level on a regular basis and communicate this information to your doctor, who will then prescribe the proper medication for pain management, if necessary. Some nurses—oncology nurses—have special expertise in treating people with cancer; however, all nurses are capable of caring for cancer patients. In the rare event that you require a permanent or temporary colostomy, a specially trained nurse called an enterostomal therapist may help you care for and adjust to this device.

Registered Dietitian

While being treated for colorectal cancer and afterward, you will have special nutritional and dietary needs since your body requires a good supply of nutrients both to fight disease and to heal from the impact of treatment. A dietitian will design a diet for you that provides adequate calories, protein, vitamins, and minerals, and will help you and your family with diet planning for the long term. If your recovery is prolonged and you cannot get enough nutrition from food, you will be put on some form of total parenteral nutrition (TPN), in which carbohydrates, protein, vitamins, and minerals are administered intravenously during your hospital stay.

Some cancer treatments, including surgery, chemotherapy, and radiation therapy, can cause problems such as chewing and swallowing difficulties, dryness in your mouth, loss of appetite, nausea or vomiting, water retention, constipation, and diarrhea. All of these can compromise the nutrition you need. A dietitian, however, can help provide strategies for overcoming the nutritional side effects of treatment. Most hospitals have registered dietitians on staff, designated by the initials *RD*.

Physical Therapist

Following surgery and other treatments, you may experience a loss of strength and feel deconditioned, even if you were relatively fit prior to treatment. A physical therapist can help you regain your strength after surgery by devising a regimen of daily walking or activity involving active or passive range-of-motion exercises. This will help strengthen your muscles, improve your joint mobility, and get you back on your feet again.

Social Worker

When dealing with cancer, you and your loved ones often feel upset, helpless, fearful, and uncertain. To help you cope, a social worker can provide counseling and a referral to group counseling or support group so that you can navigate the emotional difficulties and stress involved with a cancer diagnosis and treatment plan. He or she can also help you sort through the confusion of making treatment decisions and communicating with your doctor.

Because you may need medical assistance at home after being discharged from the hospital, your social worker can arrange for various types of assistance, including visiting nurse services, physical therapy, medical supplies and equipment, transportation, and insurance coverage.

Clergy

Many people dealing with cancer turn to their spiritual beliefs as a source of strength and hope. I find this to be extremely helpful to many of my patients. Having faith has been shown in a growing body of medical studies to improve the outcome of disease, speed recovery, and enhance the immune system. Thus, providing spiritual comfort is the all-important responsibility of the clergy as a member of the health care team. A compassionate clergy member can help you find renewed meaning in life, work through your deepest emotions and beliefs, and guide you through the difficult issues of death and afterlife. If you don't have a pastor, priest, or rabbi, then consider talking to the hospital's chaplain, who can help you with these matters, plus direct you to other clergy and worship centers in your community.

MOVE TOWARD ACTION

As you prepare to undergo treatment, there are three key actions you should take.

Get Informed

Talk to your doctor about your diagnosis, treatment options, and other issues related to your medical condition. Getting up to speed on colorectal cancer will start dissipating your negative emotions in ways you can only imagine. Some questions to ask:

- *What treatment are you recommending for me?*
- *Could you describe the treatment or procedure for me?*
- *Why are you recommending this treatment?*
- *What are the goals of this treatment?*
- *What is the success rate of this treatment?*
- *What side effects can I expect?*
- *How can these side effects be minimized or treated?*
- *What are the possible complications?*
- *How should I prepare for this treatment in order to reduce complications?*
- *What sort of follow-up care will be required?*
- *How will this treatment affect my lifestyle?*
- *What will it cost?*

The more informed you are, the better able you'll be to make appropriate decisions that are comfortable and acceptable to you, without compromising the course of your treatment. As you talk to your doctor, take notes. In addition, have a spouse, family member, friend, or other advocate by your side to make sure that you have a clear understanding of what you hear.

Get a Second Opinion

Obtaining a second opinion has become a common practice in medicine today, especially when major surgery is involved. Second opinions are useful in cases in which the diagnosis is clear, but treatment choices may vary. Some insurance plans require it. In fact, your doctor may welcome the second opinion. If your doctor is against second opinions, then, to put it bluntly, you'll need to get another doctor.

Here are some guidelines to follow when seeking a second opinion:

- Beware of shallow second opinions. Are you really getting a second opinion, or is your doctor just sending you to one of his or her colleagues in the same practice, clinic, or hospital? Make sure you get an independent evaluation from someone who is not associated with your doctor.
- Bring your medical records with you, or ask that copies be sent to the doctor rendering the second opinion. These records should include all tests, pathology slides, and reports.
- During a second-opinion conference, ask the doctor such questions as: *Why do you have this opinion? Why do you suggest this treatment? Is there anything you feel has been overlooked?*

Should the second opinion differ from the first, it might be wise to get your family doctor involved to give you advice, or ask the two doctors to explain their differences in more detail or justify the discrepancies between the two opinions. In cases like these, some insurance companies will authorize a third opinion.

Keep a Treatment Log

This lets you keep track of your personal treatment process and includes names of everyone on the treatment team, their phone numbers, an appointment calendar, the tests and procedures you've had, and an up-to-date list of the medications you're taking. By keeping a treatment log, you can provide any physician with a "snapshot" of your medical care. There is a sample treatment log in the back of this book.

As a patient, you are a key player on your health care team, with the right to monitor your own health and receive the best care possible. You always have the option to learn as much as you can about your medical condition, make informed choices about your own care, and play an active role in deciding what is best for you. You cannot change your diagnosis, but you can and should be involved in making decisions about your care and treatment—and this can go a long way toward healing and improving your quality of life.

Chapter 9

When Surgery Is the Answer

Once cancer is diagnosed, what happens next?

Answer: The operating room. After you have been diagnosed with colorectal cancer, your doctor will recommend surgery because it is considered the primary treatment for this disease and offers the best chance for a complete cure.

Surgery is the first-line treatment for stages I through III, where the major goal is to cure the cancer. Even in certain situations of stage IV disease, colon cancer may still be curable if there are isolated liver metastases that can be completely removed surgically. With more advanced stage IV colon cancer, however, surgery is not usually performed with prospect of curing the cancer, but rather to treat bowel blockages, bleeding, and perforations. For rectal cancer, your doctor may also recommend surgery, often with preoperative radiation and chemotherapy to shrink the tumor prior to surgery.

There have been amazing innovations in detection, anesthesia, antibiotics, and surgical techniques, even though the actual surgery for colorectal cancer has changed very little over the past thirty years. For colon cancer, surgeons cut out the cancerous section, along with any suspicious tissue, and reattach the two healthy segments of the colon inside the abdomen. Rarely is there a need for a colostomy, an opening from the colon to the skin of the abdomen so that stool can be eliminated into a "bag." Surgery for rectal cancer involves a different procedure, so I'll discuss both types of surgery separately in this chapter.

SURGERY AND THE STATE OF YOUR HEALTH

Prior to colon or rectal surgery, there are some important preliminaries to take care of. To begin with your surgeon will want to examine you thoroughly, review your medical history, and have you take some additional tests to pinpoint the precise location of the cancer and clinically stage the extent of the disease, as well as to decide what other treatments you may need.

Equally important, the surgeon wants to ascertain whether surgery will be safe for you. For example, the surgeon wants to know whether your heart and lungs are in good enough shape to withstand the stress of the general anesthesia used during surgery. Further, if you have a serious preexisting medical condition, you might not be able to tolerate the surgery or postoperative chemotherapy. Some examples of high-surgical-risk conditions that raise a surgeon's eyebrows include heart disease (coronary artery disease, valvular disease, and congestive heart failure), lung disease (emphysema or smoking), liver failure (cirrhosis), kidney failure, and vascular disease such as aneurysm. Any chronic or recent illness can also increase your risk of complications from the surgical procedure.

On the other hand, if you have a history of excellent health and physical activity, this may make a positive difference in how you respond to surgery. With this information, your surgeon and medical doctors will weigh the benefits of surgery against the possible risks. If you're like most patients, you are often so devastated with the news of having cancer that you say, *What good is being fit and eating right if I now have cancer?* The answer is simple: Being fit greatly improves your recovery after surgery and any post-surgical medical therapy that is needed.

Table 9-1 outlines the presurgery tests and evaluations you may have. If everything looks good, your surgeon will probably schedule you for your operation within a few days.

Table 9-1

Presurgery Tests and Evaluations

Test	Requirement	How It Works	What the Results Mean
Carcinoembryonic antigen (CEA)	Always done.	Measures a protein called CEA in the blood that in high levels is a chemical marker of cancer. Cancer cells contain CEA and release it into the blood.	High levels indicate that cancer exists. Results of this test can be used to follow and monitor the course of cancer. CEA should *never* be used for screening purposes.
Liver function blood tests	Always done.	Measures levels of liver enzymes, as well as a chemical called bilirubin that passes through the liver. Ordered because the liver is the most common site to which colorectal cancer spreads.	Excess amounts of these chemicals in the blood can indicate a tumor, blockage, or disease in the liver.
Complete blood cell count (CBC)	Always done.	Measures the number of red and white blood cells as a part of a complete health checkup.	Abnormalities may suggest anemia, infections, and blood disorders.
Chest X ray	Always done.	Helps determine whether colorectal cancer has spread to your lungs or if you suffer from other lung conditions such as emphysema.	Abnormalities pinpoint lung disorders, which may make colorectal surgery unsafe and may increase the risk of anesthesia-related complications.
Computerized tomography (CT) scans	Always done.	X ray imaging takes cross-sectional pictures of the inside of the body to look for abnormalities and monitor the course of a disease.	Images can reveal enlarged lymph nodes and metastases.
Electrocardiogram (EKG)	Always done.	A test that takes an electronic tracing of your heart in order to detect any abnormalities that could compromise anesthesia and surgery.	Abnormalities suggest heart valve dysfunction, fluid collections around the heart, heart enlargement, disease of the heart muscle, coronary artery disease, and other cardiac disorders.
Magnetic resonance imaging (MRI)	Performed only if CT scan is uncertain or if the liver needs to be better evaluated.	An imaging technique that uses powerful magnetic fields instead of X-ray radiation to display a cross section of the body.	MRI gives an accurate view and location of any growths or abnormalities that are present and is helpful in locating metastases, especially in the liver, that are sometimes difficult to see on CT scans.

Positron-emission tomography (PET) scan	Sometimes done if there is a suspicion of small metastases.	A nuclear test that measures metabolic activity.	This is a new test that may be able to show very small areas of cancer that may not be visible on other imaging techniques.
Angiography	Rarely done.	A test in which a tube is inserted into a blood vessel until it reaches the area to be viewed. A contrast dye is injected through the tube, and a series of X rays is taken.	This test pinpoints the location of blood vessels next to a liver metastasis from colorectal cancer so that the surgeon can plan the operation to minimize blood loss.
Anorectal ultrasound or Endoscopic ultrasound (EUS)	Done for some cases of rectal cancer, especially if a transanal approach is considered.	An instrument is inserted into the rectum and takes pictures with reflected sound waves (ultrasound) to see how deeply the tumor has penetrated the wall of the rectum.	The extent of tumor penetration helps determine the type of rectal surgery that is required.
Anesthesia interview	Always done.	A discussion with an anesthesiologist prior to surgery in order to minimize risks associated with anesthesia.	You'll be asked about drugs you're taking, drugs you're allergic to, and whether you've experienced any adverse side effects as a result of anesthesia in the past.

SURGERY FOR COLON CANCER

There are several different types of surgeries used to treat colon cancer, and the one that's best for you depends on many factors, including the location of your cancer and the state of your health. The main goal of most surgery, of course, is to cure the cancer by removing the tumor. As I explained in chapter 7, the pathologist's examination of the tumor and any additional tissue that is removed provides important information about whether the cancer has spread and how far. This information will be used to plan additional treatments such as chemotherapy and radiation therapy.

Before any surgical procedure is performed, your bowel needs to be prepped. This allows for a clean colon and minimizes the risk of contamination and infection by fecal matter. Two days prior to surgery, you'll be instructed to follow a specific bowel preparation using a laxative such as GoLytely/NuLytely/Colyte, or Fleet Phospho-Soda, similar to the type of prep you followed prior to a colonoscopy (see chapter 3). Taking antibiotics may be a part of your prep, too, in order to kill any harmful bacteria that may be residing in your colon.

Now for an overview of the types of surgeries performed for colon cancer.

Partial Colectomy

The most common type of operation performed for colon cancer is a partial colectomy, which removes a portion of your colon. During this operation, your surgeon makes a six- to twelve-inch incision in the middle of your abdomen to explore the abdominal cavity and remove the cancer, a margin of normal tissue around the cancer, and associated lymph nodes. In most patients, one-third of the colon is removed.

Once the section of colon is taken out, the surgeon reconnects the two healthy ends of your colon inside your abdomen in order to reconstruct the normal tubular anatomy of your gastrointestinal tract. The point of reconnection is termed the *anastomosis*.

Suturing techniques or sophisticated anatomic stapling devices are used to join the two ends together. Some patients are very concerned when they hear that their intestine is being put back together with "staples." Let me assure you, the metal staples used for the anastomosis are safe in the body, they cause no side effects, and are an excellent surgical technique to reconstruct the bowel.

Your colon is pliable, which is why it can be shortened and rejoined without really affecting your digestive system. You may experience more frequent or loose bowel movements after this surgery. This condition may come and go, but can be controlled medically.

Generally, this operation lasts between one and three hours. Normally, you can leave the hospital in five to seven days and resume your normal activities in about six weeks. The main reason that you need to remain in the hospital is that the small and large intestine become "paralyzed" temporarily after colon surgery, a condition know as an ileus. It is for this reason that your doctors will listen closely for bowel sounds and frequently ask if you are passing gas or having bowel movements. In our line of work, gastroenterologists love to hear that postoperative patients are passing gas. It's "music to our ears," and it makes us happy.

Subtotal and Total Colectomy

In a subtotal colectomy, your surgeon removes more than 90 percent of your colon. This is not a very common procedure for colon cancer; it's performed only if you have two separate colon cancers in two different parts of your colon. During this operation, ends of the remaining colon can still be reattached.

A total colectomy removes your entire colon. This is a rare procedure for cancer, however. It is usually performed in cases of familial adenomatous polyposis (FAP) as a preventive measure against the development of colon cancer, or in other medical conditions where the entire colon is diseased, as in ulcerative colitis.

So that the rectum works normally after the colon is removed, the surgeon will surgically alter the ileum (the end of the small intestine) to create a pouch that is attached to the anal sphincter muscles. This creates what is called a neo-rectum, and with time you should be able to eliminate normally, with good anal control.

Laparoscopy

Laparoscopy, also known as "keyhole" or "Band-Aid surgery," has been used for several years to treat gallbladder and gynecologic problems, but now it is being used increasingly in colorectal and other forms of gastrointestinal surgery.

In laparoscopic surgery, your abdomen is inflated with a harmless gas through a small "keyhole" incision at your belly button. The gas lifts your abdomen away from the other organs so that the surgeon can better view the site. The surgeon then inserts a thin, telescope-like instrument called a laparoscope through the incision. The laparoscope is connected to a video camera no bigger than a dime, and the camera projects the view of your abdominal cavity onto television screens in the operating room. The surgeon operates by passing small surgical instruments through one or more additional incisions. When the surgery is completed, the gas is released from your abdomen, and the incisions are closed up. The benefits of laparoscopy are less pain after surgery, a shorter hospital stay (one or two days), less scarring, less suppression of your immune system, and a faster return to your normal activities.

Currently, most experts accept laparoscopy as an effective technique to remove malignant polyps and early-stage cancer. But we still do not know if laparoscopic surgery is as good as conventional surgery for treating more advanced stages of cancer.

Realistically, laparoscopy is not suitable for everyone. If you have conditions such as obesity; advanced kidney, lung, or heart disease; or previous abdominal surgeries, this procedure may not be right for you. Talk to your surgeon about whether or not you are a good candidate for laparoscopic surgery.

SURGERY FOR RECTAL CANCER

Surgeons use a variety of techniques to remove a rectal tumor, ranging from radical procedures to newer techniques that preserve the anal sphincter muscles. Keeping the sphincter muscles intact eliminates the need for a colostomy. Here is a look at the types of procedures performed for rectal surgery.

Low Anterior Resection (LAR)

The most common abdominal surgery used to treat rectal cancers, regardless of stage, is a low anterior resection, in which cancer located in the lower one-third of the sigmoid colon or upper two-thirds of the rectum is taken out. During this operation, your surgeon will make a vertical incision in the center of your abdomen in order to remove the cancer and adjacent lymph nodes. Once these tissues are removed, your colon is attached to the lower half of the rectum, and you can eliminate waste in the normal way. You will recover in the hospital for at least a week.

Transanal Excision

Some early-stage rectal tumors or polyps that are located close to the anus but have not yet invaded the inner lining of the rectum (stage T_1 or less) can be removed through the anus without entering the abdominal cavity. This procedure is called a transanal excision.

Prior to surgery, an anorectal ultrasound or endoscopic ultrasound (EUS) is performed by a gastroenterologist or surgeon. In either procedure a small ultrasound probe is placed in the rectum to evaluate the depth of penetration of the tumor into the rectal wall and to look for abnormally large lymph nodes. Some surgeons will proceed directly to the operating room to perform a transanal excision based on their digital (finger) examination. In the present era of rectal surgery, however, you should insist on an ultrasound if transanal surgery is being considered. Only ultrasound can accurately determine the depth of tumor penetration into the rectal wall. Following ultrasound staging to determine the appropriateness of transanal excision, your surgeon will remove the tumor and a margin of normal rectum.

Advantages of transanal excision include dramatically less trauma to your body, less physical pain, and no colostomy. What's more, this procedure can be performed on an outpatient basis, although some patients may need to stay overnight in the hospital. Because lymph nodes are not removed in this operation, you may require chemotherapy and radiation therapy afterward to kill any cancer cells that may remain in your body. It is important to mention that this is a highly specialized operation that should be performed by a colorectal cancer surgeon with advanced training and experience in this technique.

Abdominoperineal Resection (APR)

The most extensive surgery for rectal cancer is an abdominoperineal resection, used for cancers in the lower part of the rectum, close to its connection to the anus. It involves removing the lower end of the rectum and anus, and usually the creation of a permanent colostomy (see below). If the anal sphincter muscles can be spared, there is a possibility that a colostomy can be avoided. Once again, this decision needs to be made by a skilled colorectal cancer surgeon. You'll have to stay in the hospital for about a week following this operation.

COLOSTOMY

In rare cases in which the surgeon is unable to reconnect the sections of your bowel, a temporary or permanent colostomy may be necessary. Colostomy is a surgical procedure that makes an opening, called a stoma, in your abdominal wall through which a small part of the colon is routed to the surface of your skin. Stool passes through this opening and empties directly into an external bag, or pouch. This pouch sticks to your skin with a special glue. It does not show under your clothes, and it is easy for most people to take care of by themselves. While you are in the hospital, an enterostomal therapist will show you how to select a pouching system that is right for you, as well as how to care for your colostomy. With a colostomy in place, you no longer have voluntary control over your bowel movements, and you must familiarize yourself with the frequency of your elimination and bowel habits.

Normally, a colostomy is only temporary, put in place to allow time for your bowel to heal. After healing has occurred, your surgeon will remove the colostomy and rejoin the two sections of the bowel. Once this happens, your digestive functions will get back to normal.

You'll require a colostomy if the colon cancer is so large that it completely obstructs your colon. In a case like this, the colon cannot be evacuated with a bowel prep prior to surgery. Thus, a colostomy will be created so that stool can pass and be eliminated freely. This procedure is called a diverting colostomy, and it is usually temporary. At a later date, the colon will be reattached, and the colostomy removed.

The colostomy may be permanent, however, in some late-stage cancers and for rectal cancer located close to the anus that involves the anal sphincter muscles. For the small number of people who require one, the thought of a colostomy is as overwhelming as having cancer. Even so, it is not as bad as people imagine. Given the choice of life or colostomy, trust me when I say that I have never had a patient regret living!

Having a colostomy does not have to change your life nor make it any less meaningful. Quite the contrary; you can continue to enjoy all your normal activities of working, traveling, enjoying intimate relationships, swimming, exercising, and playing sports. Fortunately, the number of colostomies needed is dropping, thanks to early detection and improved surgical procedures.

METASTATIC CANCER: IF YOUR CANCER HAS SPREAD TO THE LIVER

If cancer has spread to your liver your surgeon may recommend an operation to remove the metastases. Removing these tumors can sometimes cure the cancer, or help a patient live longer. Any surgical approach to metastatic disease is also combined with chemotherapy. This is discussed in the next chapter.

The preferred surgical procedure is a partial liver resection in which the tumor(s) and a margin of normal liver tissue are removed. If surgical resection is not possible for anatomic or medical reasons, then ablative therapies utilizing freezing or heating may be the best option. Cryosurgery destroys the tumor by freezing it, and thermal ablation removes it by heating it with microwaves or radio frequencies. The surgeon inserts the freezing probe or microwave probe through your skin and guides it to the tumor using a CT scan or ultrasound.

If cancer has spread to the liver and surgery is not an option, the surgeon may elect to surgically implant a hepatic artery pump into the liver so that it can be directly infused with chemotherapy. This will also be discussed more thoroughly in the next chapter.

RECURRENT COLORECTAL CANCER

Recurrent colorectal cancer is cancer that returns after you have been successfully treated and have enjoyed a period free of any detectable cancer. With recurrent colorectal cancer, surgery (in addition to chemotherapy) remains an important part of the primary treatment if cancer returns at the anastomosis site (where the colon was rejoined), or if new metastases occur in the liver.

The surgical strategy always depends on the type of recurrence. For example, if cancer appears in the anastomosis, this area will be surgically removed, and a new anastomosis will be created. If the cancer has spread into the lining of the abdominal cavity, called carcinomatosis, some doctors will recommend surgery to remove as much of the tumor's bulk as possible, followed by chemotherapy infused directly into the abdomen (a procedure known as intraperitoneal chemotherapy). This therapy is controversial, and should be considered experimental.

Because of the possibility of recurrence, you should remain ever vigilant regarding your health, report any changes or unusual symptoms to your doctor, and stick religiously to the follow-up and screening strategies outlined by your doctor. In chapter 12, I will discuss how recurrences are monitored.

THE POTENTIAL COMPLICATIONS OF SURGERY

All surgery carries with it the risk of complications, and colorectal surgery is no exception. The good news, however, is that major complications following colorectal surgery are relatively rare, occurring in less than 5 percent of patients. But you do need to be aware of which complications could arise, since many are life threatening if not treated immediately. Some of the major complications of colorectal surgery are:

- An adverse reaction to general anesthesia.
- Abdominal bleeding.
- Infections. These may include intrabdominal abscess (there is more risk of this with rectal cancer than with colon cancer); pneumonia; wound infection; and urinary tract infection.
- Blood clots in the legs (with potential migration to the lungs, called a pulmonary embolus).
- A possible heart attack.
- Bowel leakage.

- A fistula (an abnormal connection between the skin and intestine that can cause stool to leak out, leading to an infection).
- Injury to other organs.

PREPARING FOR SURGERY

You can minimize the risk of complications considerably and maximize your chances of having a successful operation by adequately preparing for surgery. What I do with my patients to help ensure a complication-free operation is to have them prepare a checklist prior to surgery. Here is an example.

A Checklist of Everything to Do Prior to Surgery

- Stop taking prescription and over-the-counter medications that interfere with blood clotting at least seven days prior to surgery. These include such drugs as aspirin, Naprosyn (Aleve), and ibuprofen (Motrin and Advil). If you are unsure about whether a medication causes this side effect, check with your doctor.
- If you are on blood-thinning medications such as Coumadin, discuss with your cardiologist or hematologist when to take your last dose before surgery.
- Stop taking certain vitamins and herbal preparations at least seven days prior to surgery. Vitamin E, *Ginkgo biloba,* kava, ginger, saw palmetto, garlic pills, and feverfew are examples of dietary supplements that can interact with anesthesia or thin your blood, increasing the risk of surgical complications. Make sure your surgeon and nurses know about every medication or supplement you are taking.
- Designate a friend or family member as your advocate, to talk to your surgeon following your operation and to communicate with your other physicians about your outcome.
- Check your company's health and disability benefits by contacting the human resources department, and have a meeting with your supervisor regarding your sick leave, and when you

might be expected to return to work. If you feel comfortable discussing your illness with your employer, this may help alleviate the stress, worry, and uncertainty that can arise over employment issues. If you are self-employed, make sure your disability insurance pays your salary while you're not working.

- Arrange your work schedule so that someone can fill in for you while you are away, and let your supervisor and coworkers know how long you expect to be off.

- Recruit help. Arrange for someone to take care of your household tasks while you are hospitalized.

- Carefully follow your surgeon's bowel preparation instructions. Doing so will help minimize the risk of infection and improve your surgical outcome.

- Bank your own blood if you are overly concerned about getting a bloodborne disease from a blood transfusion. Personally, I do not recommend this, because the risk of receiving tainted blood is extremely low—less than 0.01 percent. However, if you decide that you want to bank your own blood, self-donation is relatively easy and may help alleviate some of your fears. If you are already anemic or the surgery is going to be performed soon, blood donation will not be possible. In such cases, you may consider having a friend or family member with the same blood type donate specifically for you. You can check with your surgeon about whether you may require a blood transfusion and how you can stockpile your own blood in the event that you might need one.

- Stop smoking and using recreational drugs. These increase your risk of complications. Smoking, in particular, affects anesthesia and increases the possibility of lung complications during surgery. Quitting smoking prior to surgery, even for a short duration of time, can improve your outcome. From surgery to wound healing to postoperative recovery, not smoking will improve your overall ability to heal.

- Stop drinking alcohol. Drinking even a glass or two of wine or beer (or more than a shot of hard liquor) daily can interfere with the effects of anesthesia.

RECOVERING SUCCESSFULLY FROM SURGERY

After spending a week or less in the hospital, if all goes well, your doctor will announce the good news that you can now go home. What this means is that you'll spend four to eight weeks recovering at home. It is all-important that you follow your doctor's instructions to the letter, so that you can bounce back successfully following surgery. Here's what to do for the healthiest recovery possible, both in the hospital and at home.

Pain Management

While in the hospital, you will experience pain, mostly from the incision. To relieve the pain, you'll be given pain medication, based on how you rate the severity of your pain.

Even after returning home, you may still be in pain. However, this should last no more than four or five days. Pain can cause undue exhaustion and stress, which can interfere with healing, so use the pain-relieving medication prescribed by your doctor; don't try to grit your teeth and get through it. If your pain should increase, however, notify your surgeon at once. There are numerous ways to manage pain in addition to medication, and these are discussed in chapter 11. They include complementary therapies that enhance effective pain management.

Caring for Incisions

Your incision will usually begin to heal about one to two days after your surgery, and often the dressings will be removed by your nurse to let the air circulation enhance the healing of the wound. Don't be scared if you still see staples! These often remain in place until after discharge from the hospital. They will be painlessly removed by the surgeon or assistant when you return to the office for your checkup. Once you get home, follow your doctor's instructions for changing dressings and bandages. When showering, gently wash around your incision, using mild unscented soap. Don't take a bath until your wound fully closes.

Be sure to watch for signs of infection related to the incision. These include redness, swelling, and drainage. Get in touch with your surgeon immediately if you notice any of these signs.

Diet

After surgery, you'll be given a liquid diet for a few days, a regimen consisting of liquids you can see through, such as broth, Jell-O, and apple juice. At around the fourth day of your hospital stay, once you start passing gas or having bowel movements, you'll advance to soft foods such as soups and applesauce. These diets give your intestines time to rest and heal without unnecessary strain and irritation.

Prior to leaving the hospital, you should meet with a dietitian to go over important nutrition issues. Once you get home, you should stick to what is known as a low-residue diet. This is essentially a soft foods diet with very little fiber, consisting of cooked fruits and vegetables, soups, ice cream, yogurt, and nutritional beverages and puddings such as Boost or Ensure. Eating too much fiber at this stage of recovery could irritate your colon, so you have to be careful. You should stay on a low-residue diet for a few weeks.

After your doctor's evaluation of your progress, you should be able to advance to a more normal diet in which you slowly increase your fiber intake. Gradually start eating fresh fruits, vegetables, and whole grains, adjusting the amount according to how these foods affect your digestion. Be sure to drink at least eight glasses of water a day to keep yourself well hydrated and help ward off postsurgery constipation that can result from both pain medications and a lack of exercise.

Breathing Exercises

After your surgery, either your nurses or a respiratory therapist will encourage you to practice deep breathing and coughing. This helps prevent atelectasis, in which the tiny air sacs in your lungs collapse due to shallow breathing. Symptoms include shortness of breath, cough, and fever. Atelectasis can be prevented if you are up and walking around as soon as possible. You will also be encouraged to take deep breaths to expand the lungs and blow on a device called an incentive spirometer to encourage rapid, forceful breathing. At first, deep breathing may hurt, so start slowly and work on the incentive spirometer until you can tolerate the deeper breaths.

Don't be afraid to use the prescribed pain medication, either. This is important not only for your comfort, but also for allowing deep breaths. The incentive spirometer can help you expand your lungs, and you should use it often.

Continue to do your breathing exercises even after you have returned home. In addition to breathing, try to gently cough once or twice in order to loosen mucus and other secretions that may have built up in your lungs.

Exercise

The best activity you can do following surgery is walking. Too much bed rest after surgery is dangerous because it can lead to deep-vein thrombosis, the formation of a blood clot deep within the leg. This blood clot can travel to your lungs and may create a very serious condition known as a pulmonary embolus.

Walking also helps normalize your digestive system, eases pain, prevents lung collapse, and enhances overall healing. Beginning shortly after surgery in the hospital and continuing when you return home, begin to walk short distances. Try to increase the distance when you feel up to it. Do not try to do too much; listen to your body and to your energy levels. Walk when you feel like it; rest when you don't. But do try to walk every day.

In the days and weeks following your surgery, you'll feel like your get-up-and-go has got up and gone. That's natural and to be expected. But rest assured that your strength and stamina will begin to return shortly after your discharge from the hospital. It may take time, and your energy level may fluctuate. Some days, you may feel quite energetic; on others, your fatigue may be overwhelming. Again, these highs and lows are completely normal.

Please consult your surgeon about the appropriate postsurgical exercise regimen for you. In particular, your surgeon will advise you to avoid lifting because it puts too much strain on your abdominal muscles. Nor should you do any sit-ups, push-ups, bending, or stretching until your surgeon gives you the go-ahead.

Bowel Management

In about 20 percent of patients who have surgery for colorectal cancer, there is a change in bowel habits. If your sigmoid colon was removed, for example, you may notice softer, more frequent bowel movements. If your rectum was removed, you may have more frequent and urgent bowel movements. At times, you may feel as if your bowel hasn't been totally emptied.

Generally, these problems develop because surgery alters the anatomical structure of your colon or rectum, or both. If a large part of your colon was removed, you will probably require medication such as Imodium (now available over the counter) or Lomotil (a prescription drug) to slow the movement of material through your intestine and colon. If the right side of your colon was removed, along with the valve that connects the small intestine to the large intestine (known as the ileocecal valve), you may have a type of diarrhea caused by bile salts, which act like a digestive detergent to break down fats and oils into smaller droplets. The ileocecal valve works as an intestinal "brake," when it's absent, the small intestinal contents pour rapidly into the colon. These bile salts, which are normally reabsorbed by the small intestine, may enter your colon and can cause diarrhea. A resin-based medication called cholestyramine (Questran) binds with bile salts and dramatically improves the diarrhea. Ask your doctor about this medication if you had right-sided colon surgery.

If only a small part of your colon or rectum was removed, especially in the sigmoid or rectum, you may need to retrain the way your colon functions. To assist with this readjustment, you may need to follow a bowel management program to resolve these problems and protect the health of your colon and rectum. Okay, you're probably scratching your head right now, wondering, *A bowel management program? What is that all about?*

Actually, it's the adult version of potty training—a way to improve your bowel habits and condition your colon to act as nature intended. Your bowel does not know that a piece of it is missing, and its timing may be off with regard to regular bowel habits. Training your bowel to become more regular may not sound like much fun to you right now, and it's true that bowel problems are no laughing matter, but try to maintain your sense of humor and you'll do a great job of answering nature's call. Here are some general guidelines to help you:

Control Peristalsis

Normally, eating a large meal or drinking a hot liquid stimulates peristalsis (the muscular contractions of the digestive system), thereby pushing material more rapidly through your system. But if you're having too-frequent bowel movements, you must slow this process down. The easiest way to do this is to drink less fluid with your meals and steer clear of hot liquids just before, during, or right after mealtime.

Slow Down Transit Time

If it feels like you're camping out in the bathroom due to frequent bowel movements, take a fiber supplement such as Metamucil, Citrucel, or FiberCon tablets. Normally, these supplements help clear up constipation and accelerate bowel transit time, but they can also be used to slow it down, if used in the following manner:

After you eat a meal, take the prescribed amount of the supplement (about a teaspoon) with very little liquid. Don't drink any fluid for one hour after that meal. This allows the fiber in the supplement to soak up any excess fluid in your digestive tract, and will put the brakes on your transit time. Do this at the same meal for three to five days, or until your transit time slows down and normalizes. Be aware, however, that this may also increase the amount of gas in your system, especially when you first add fiber.

Bowel-Train Yourself

The goal of "bowel training" is to empty your colon fully at a certain time each day. Begin your bowel-training program after your stools have become better formed and your transit time has slowed down. There are usually five steps involved, although these may vary from doctor to doctor:

- Because the most natural time to use the toilet is after a meal, pick a large meal around which you'll bowel-train yourself. Large meals are best, since they activate the movement response of your intestines.
- Eat your meal.
- Drink a hot liquid.
- Sit on the toilet about half an hour after the meal, even if you do not feel like you have to have a bowel movement. If you have the urge to move your bowels before this time, go to the bathroom sooner.
- Follow this mealtime procedure for three days in a row. If it does not produce results—that is, the planned emptying of your bowels—you may want to use a suppository after drinking the hot liquid in order to stimulate a complete bowel movement. Your doctor can advise you on which type of suppository to use.

If this five-step training program works, continue the regimen for two weeks. After the two-week period is up, discontinue using the suppositories. The large meal and the hot liquid should be all your body needs in order to fully empty your bowel.

Because everyone is different, you may have to adjust your bowel management program, with assistance from your doctor or other health care professionals. You may have to take antidiarrhea medicine such as Imodium, Lomotil, or other medications as discussed above. Whatever your particular situation, bowel management involves balancing your food, fluid intake, fiber, and medication. Just be patient, work with your doctor or nurse, and your bowel function should improve.

Probiotic Therapy

One important bowel intervention after surgery that your doctor may not tell you about is probiotic therapy. Probiotics are friendly bacteria, such as those found in yogurt, that in my experience seem to improve the colon's ability to heal and function normally. In fact, most of my patients report a significant improvement in bowel habits with probiotic usage during the period they are recovering from surgery.

The best strains of probiotics for the colon include *Lactobacillus* (my personal favorite is *Lactobacillus GG,* sold as Culterelle), *Bifidobacterium bifidum, Saccharomyces boulardii* (sold as Floraster), and a friendly version of *E. Coli* (sold as Probactrix). A good combination of probiotics is available in a product called VSL#3. Depending on what product you use, follow the label instructions for correct dosage. Web sites for these probiotics are provided in "Resources."

Sexual Side Effects

Sometimes men and women may experience sexual problems following treatment for colorectal cancer. Most cancer survivors are not prepared for changes in their sex lives.

When you feel like your life is hanging in the balance, you may understandably put the need for sex at the bottom of your priority list. This reaction is perfectly normal and is shared by many people after treatment for colorectal cancer. The stress of facing a life-threatening diagnosis, followed by the pain and fatigue that results from surgery and chemotherapy, can exact a toll on your body image, your feelings of sexiness, and your energy level.

There may be physical reasons for sexual problems as well. Both surgery and radiation can interfere with the sacral nerves located at the base of your spine. These nerves are involved in sexual function and can be compromised when surgery removes cancer from a low section of your colon or rectum. In men, radiation to the pelvic area can inflict damage on the blood vessels required to achieve an erection.

Although it may be uncomfortable for you, for your doctor, or both to bring up these issues, try to be open and honest about your concerns, because there is a wide range of treatments that can help restore normal sexual activity, especially for men.

To put your mind at ease, let me reassure you that you can still enjoy sex and intimacy after treatment for colorectal cancer. The most important aspect of regaining intimacy is the feeling that you want to reconnect with your partner and move forward. For starters, reestablish your "chemistry" by doing the things that have always been special in your relationship. This may be as simple as a quiet dinner or watching a favorite movie. Next, try creating a sensual mood for intimacy with lighting, music, or clothes you feel comfortable in. Finally, relax and just enjoy your partner's company. Remember that any approach to improved intimacy may help you regain a pleasurable sex life.

Returning to Work

It is difficult to estimate when you will be able to return to work, since every patient is different. Some are back on the job within four to six weeks of surgery, while others may require a longer period of time. If your doctor has recommended chemotherapy or radiation therapy following surgery, you may need to return to work on a part-time basis, depending on how you tolerate these treatments. The point is to not rush into anything by returning to work before you are physically and emotionally ready. Just take your time, and let yourself fully heal. Most people are able to eventually return to their jobs, successfully and with full productivity.

To ease your anxiety level over having surgery, keep in mind that surgery is the best way to cure colorectal cancer, and focusing on this will help you maintain a positive attitude. To further calm your mind and reduce stress, talk to your friends, family, clergy, and treatment team members about your feelings; use some of the mind–body techniques discussed in chapter 11; or seek spiritual comfort and guidance from your faith.

If nothing else, try to maintain your sense of humor throughout this, since humor has a healing effect on your entire body, physically and emotionally.

For many people, the prospect of having an operation is much less upsetting than being told they have cancer. After you come to grips with the diagnosis, your thinking becomes less cloudy and more focused. You accept the fact that something is wrong in your body—and that by deciding to have surgery, you're doing something to beat it.

Chapter 10

If You Need Chemotherapy or Radiation Therapy

Despite surgery's powerful ability to cure colorectal cancer, sometimes your doctor has to use chemotherapy to destroy any cancer cells that might remain in your body. Chemotherapy involves the use of anticancer drugs given intravenously or orally. These drugs go through your bloodstream and kill cancer cells.

For many of you, chemotherapy is a scary proposition because it brings to mind sick, debilitated cancer patients. It is true that chemotherapy—as one of my patients put it—is not for wimps. But let me assure you: You *can* get through it. The world of chemotherapy is rapidly changing, thanks to exciting new drugs that are better tolerated, with far fewer side effects. In fact, some of these new drugs are not "chemotherapy" at all, but instead belong to a new class of agents known as *targeted therapy*. They arrest cancer by disrupting the cellular signals that drive its out-of-control growth. Unlike chemotherapy, which attacks all dividing cells—normal *and* cancerous—targeted therapies go after the abnormalities that are distinct to the specific cancer being treated. Some agents are antibodies, which are proteins produced by immune system cells and released into the blood to defend the body against foreign agents. Anticancer antibodies target cancer cells and the blood vessels that supply them. Targeted therapies are relatively new on the scene and are mostly experimental.

Please know, too, that not everyone being treated for colorectal cancer will require chemotherapy. Whether you need additional treatment depends on whether the cancer has broken through the colon wall, if lymph nodes contain cancer, or if other organs are involved. Treatment goals are taken into consideration as well. For example, your doctor may wish to use chemotherapy to shrink a tumor prior to surgery, to destroy any cancer cells that may have migrated from the original site, or to prevent the return of cancer.

Using his or her knowledge and expertise, your doctor will design and individualize a plan of treatment just for you, based on many different factors, including the stage of your cancer, its location, how the cancer is affecting your normal bodily functions, and the state of your overall health. For stage I and stage II cancers, surgery is usually all that is required, unless tests reveal that the cancer has spread. Unfortunately, though, most colorectal cancers are not caught in an early stage.

If your cancer has metastasized, or spread, chemotherapy will almost always be a part of your plan of care, because it infiltrates your entire system to help control the growth of cancer cells. Research shows that chemotherapy increases both survival time and quality of life in late-stage colorectal cancer.

When planning treatment for rectal cancer, your doctor may consider radiation therapy, which employs radiation directed at the cancer site to eradicate the tumor. If radiation is used to treat rectal cancer, chemotherapy is also required. In this chapter, I will talk to you about radiation as well.

A major goal of chemotherapy, radiation therapy, or both is to drive your cancer into remission—a period of time when the cancer responds well to treatment, or is under control. With a complete remission, all the signs and symptoms of cancer have disappeared. When a complete remission lasts for more than five years, a patient is usually considered cured. A patient can also have a partial remission, meaning that the cancer shrinks but does not go away completely. If cancer returns, further treatment can bring it into another remission.

Let's move on to talking about the specifics of chemotherapy and radiation therapy.

ADJUVANT THERAPY FOR COLON CANCER

After you have surgery, the tissue removed is examined to find out whether your cancer has spread, and how far—in other words, to identify its stage, as described in chapter 7. Imaging tests such as CT scans can also help determine whether the cancer has progressed. If it has spread, adjuvant (meaning "additional") therapy will be given to finish off any remaining cancer cells, helping to ensure that you are cancer-free. But if you have stage I colon cancer (in which the cancer is confined to the submucosa of the colon), there's no need for chemotherapy because you run a very low risk of having your cancer return.

In stage II colon cancer (in which the cancer has spread through the muscular layer of the colon), chemotherapy may or may not be used. It is beneficial if the tumor has been staged as $T_4 N_0$, where the cancer has spread completely through the wall of the colon into nearby organs or tissues. Using chemotherapy for a $T_3 N_0$ cancer, in which the tumor has only penetrated the muscular layer of the colon wall, is still considered controversial, and doctors don't yet know whether it is effective or not.

If any lymph nodes are affected (stage III), then your doctor will most likely recommend adjuvant chemotherapy. It is used to help eradicate tumor cells too small to be seen, to prevent the recurrence of cancer, and to improve the cure rate. In stage III disease, chemotherapy can reduce the risk of recurrence following surgery by 41 percent, and it can reduce the death rate by 33 percent. Various types of chemotherapy agents are used, usually in specific combinations, and these drugs are discussed later in this chapter.

Adjuvant radiation therapy for colon cancer is rarely recommended.

ADJUVANT THERAPY FOR RECTAL CANCER

Normally with stage II or stage III rectal cancer, chemotherapy is still the primary treatment. However, radiation therapy is added to reduce the risk of recurrence in the pelvis, because rectal cancer is more likely than colon cancer to spread locally, as well as to distant organs and tissues. Radiation therapy thus helps prevent the spread and the recurrence of rectal cancer. It does not confer this benefit in colon cancer, however, and therefore is rarely used.

NEOADJUVANT THERAPY

The term *neoadjuvant therapy* refers to treatment given before surgery, usually to shrink a tumor so that it is easier to remove, or to help control tumor spread and growth.

This form of treatment is used more frequently to treat rectal cancer and employs a combination of chemo- and radiation therapy. Some doctors believe that this approach can help spare the rectum by shrinking the tumor enough so that the patient doesn't have to have a colostomy, although there is no proof of this hypothesis. What's more, some patients are able to tolerate neoadjuvant therapy better than adjuvant (treatment after surgery) therapy because they are not yet weakened by surgery.

Neoadjuvant therapy is used less often in colon cancer, because surgery may offer a total cure. In cases of advanced colon cancer that has spread to distant sites, neoadjuvant therapy may be employed to shrink the borders of a tumor prior to surgery or to reduce the size of tumors that have spread to the liver so that they may be removed in their entirety.

PALLIATIVE THERAPY

The term *palliative therapy* (or *palliative care*) refers to treatments—including surgery, chemotherapy, radiation therapy, and pain medications—that are provided not to cure the cancer, but to help relieve cancer pain and symptoms. In addition, palliative therapy may be used to help shrink a tumor, slow its growth in the body, and improve quality of life.

Telling a patient that a cure is not likely or that cancer treatment is failing is one of the most difficult discussions that a doctor can have with a patient. Despite the advances made in the treatment of colorectal cancer, sadly we still do not have the answer for everyone.

A patient who has fought the good fight against cancer may discover that the battle—at least the physical battle—is not to be won. If you or a loved one has undergone treatment for colorectal cancer and are facing the possibility that a cure is unlikely, please know that this is understandably a difficult time and whatever choices you make should be those that are right for you. In this situation, some patients may wish to consider a clinical trial—a study in which experimental drugs are tested as possible treatments for colorectal cancer. At the end of this chapter I have included information on how to apply for and participate in a clinical trial. Other patients may decide that they have endured enough therapies and side effects, and they wish to live the rest of their life in as much comfort as possible. Please remember, if you choose to forego further curative treatment for your cancer, this does not mean your doctor and other health professionals are no longer there to help you. On the contrary, we are here to help you in your journey through life, including the end of life. It is here that palliative therapy—in the form of hospice care—is helpful to many patients and their families.

The term *hospice* is a scary one to hear. It means that the cancer cannot be cured and life expectancy is usually less than six months. There are in-patient hospices as well as visiting home hospice services that focus on end-of-life palliation. Specially trained health professionals use palliative therapies to provide day-to-day care and comfort for the patient and his or her family.

Let me tell you about Calvary Hospital, a hospital/hospice in the Bronx that has been dedicated to caring for terminal cancer patients for over a hundred years.

When you enter the building, there is a banner on the main wall that reads, A PLACE WHERE LIFE CONTINUES . . . Dr. Michael Brescia, Calvary's executive director, tells patients that Calvary will "restore" them. What a wonderful way to describe the function of an institution dedicated to palliative care! Dr. Brescia cannot cure the cancer, but he can restore the dignity, humanity, and general essence of any individual in the end stages of incurable cancer. In addition, this restoration extends to the family as well since they can be assured that their loved one will be comfortable, cared for, and cared about. In fact, I know one secret ingredient in Calvary's restoration recipe: Dr. Brescia personally hugs and kisses his patients. That's right—he believes that for patients with incurable cancer who are approaching the end of their life, pure compassion is an essential part of their restoration—and I couldn't agree more. I just wish we put more emphasis on compassion in every aspect of medical care.

MEDICINES USED IN CHEMOTHERAPY

Whether you have chemotherapy before or after surgery, there are specific anticancer agents and combinations of agents that are used to treat cancer. Here is a brief rundown of each chemotherapy drug, along with a look at several agents now being investigated for their potential use in the battle against colorectal cancer.

5-Fluorouracil (5-FU, Adrucil)

For more than forty years, 5-fluorouracil has been the cornerstone chemotherapy agent for treating colorectal cancer. A member of a class of drugs known as antimetabolites, 5-fluorouracil interferes with cellular nucleic acids (DNA and RNA), which govern cell reproduction, and thus disrupts the growth of metabolically active cancer cells. It is usually given with other drugs, such as leucovorin, that help it work better. In addition, 5-fluorouracil is administered with radiation therapy to treat rectal cancer and enhance the effectiveness of the radiation.

Administered intravenously, 5-fluorouracil is slowly injected into a vein over a five-minute period. Some doctors employ a schedule of once-a-week injections. In some instances, 5-fluorouracil is given as a continuous infusion into a vein. You wear a small battery-powered pump that continuously releases the drug into an IV line. No additional chemotherapy is administered while you recover from the drug's side effects.

If the cancer has spread to your liver, 5-fluorouracil or a related drug, floxuridine (FUDR), may be infused directly to the artery that supplies blood to your liver. This method of treating metastatic colorectal cancer is called hepatic artery infusion. Unfortunately, this method of treatment may cause liver and stomach toxicity— a serious side effect that does not occur with the conventional 5-fluorouracil infusion described above.

Generally, 5-fluorouracil is well tolerated, though it may cause diarrhea, mouth sores, rash, loss of appetite, and fatigue. Fortunately, 5-FU does not cause hair loss, a common side effect of many chemotherapeutic agents.

Leucovorin (Citrovorum Factor, FA)

Leucovorin is not technically a chemotherapy drug, but rather a vitamin related to folic acid, a B vitamin, Leucovorin enhances the power of 5-fluorouracil to kill cancer cells. It's administered intravenously, or taken orally as a pill.

Side effects are rare, but may include rash and itching.

Irinotecan (Camptosar)

Irinotecan is a member of a group of drugs known as topoisomerase inhibitors. These drugs block the growth of cancer cells by halting the activity of enzymes necessary for cell division.

Irinotecan may be used alone or combined with 5-fluorouracil and other agents. It is typically used for treating metastatic colorectal cancer. Administered intravenously, the combination of irinotecan with 5-fluorouracil and leucovorin has been shown to significantly prolong survival and delay tumor growth in patients with metastatic colorectal cancer.

Diarrhea, fatigue, hair loss, and appetite changes are some of irinotecan's side effects.

Oxaliplatin (Eloxatin)

Oxaliplatin is a new platinum-based drug that belongs to a general group of drugs known as alkylating agents. An IV drug, oxaliplatin works on the DNA of cancer cells, causing them to become "sticky" and, as a result, self-destruct.

In combination therapy, oxaliplatin is used with 5-fluorouracil and leucovorin for treating advanced colon or rectal cancer where the disease has recurred or progressed during or within six months of completing therapy with 5-fluorouracil, leucovorin, and irinotecan. Some oncologists are now using 5-FU and oxaliplatin as initial front-line therapy in advanced disease.

The most common side effects of oxaliplatin are allergic reactions, numbness, tingling, sensitivity of your hands to cold, and a choking sensation when drinking cold beverages.

Capecitabine (Xeloda)

Another type of antimetabolite, capecitabine is converted into 5-fluorouracil in the body preferentially by cancer cells. In two clinical trials, capecitabine shrank metastatic colorectal tumors more effectively than the standard treatment (5-fluorouracil and leucovorin). It did not, however, produce a decrease in side effects or overall increase in survival.

The beauty of this drug is that it is taken as a pill, so you don't have to undergo intravenous chemotherapy treatment. That means less time spent at a clinic or hospital, the flexibility of taking your medication on the go, and a better quality of life during treatment. Normally, you take two pills, twelve hours apart, within 30 minutes after meals and with plenty of water.

Capecitabine's most serious side effects are diarrhea and painful redness and swelling in your hands and feet. This swelling can be soothed and controlled by taking a prescription-strength anti-inflammatory drug.

Capecitabine, technically known as an oral oncology therapy, represents a huge improvement over intravenous chemotherapy. Still, there are barriers to the widespread use of oral oncology therapies, including concerns about patient compliance and reimbursement. Patients may not take all the medicine they should, they may not take it on schedule, and they may not tell their doctors about any side effects they're experiencing. What's more, some oral medications are not affordable because insurance companies are not yet paying for them. As a result of these issues, the use of oral cancer agents has been limited.

THE NEXT GENERATION OF CANCER MEDICINES

Many other agents for colorectal cancer are being studied, including targeted therapies, different combinations of drugs, and novel ways of administering them. Let's first look at some of the exciting and promising targeted therapy agents now under investigation in clinical trials.

Avastin (anti-VEGF)

This remarkable new drug is an antibody that blocks a signal factor known as vascular endothelial growth factor (VEGF, pronounced, *VEG-ef*). In doing so, this drug kills a tumor by altering its blood supply. Specifically, it normalizes the structure of blood vessels and stops tumors from building blood vessels. Consequently, the cancer cells do not get an adequate blood supply and they die. Avastin represents the first class of anticancer drugs that exert this action.

Now in progress are studies to determine whether Avastin is ready for widespread use. So far, scientists have learned that the drug works better in smaller doses, rather than larger ones, and that it significantly improves survival when combined with irinotecan-based chemotherapy in the first-line treatment of metastatic colon cancer.

When added to standard irinotecan-based therapy, Avastin prolonged survival by approximately five months. This exciting finding has generated a lot of attention and research utilizing this new agent. Avastin may be available by the time you read this book.

Its side effects include blood clots, high blood pressure, and nosebleeds.

Erbitux (Cetuximab or C-225)

Now being studied in many different cancers, including colon cancer, cetuximab is an example of a monoclonal antibody, a new group of drugs that can locate tumor cells and either kill them or deliver tumor-killing substances to them without harming normal cells. Administered intravenously, cetuximab blocks the receptor, or signal, for a growth factor called epidermal growth factor (EGF) on the surface of cells. By interfering with this signal, cell growth is stopped, and tumor growth is thus interrupted. EGF-receptor-targeted therapies are being investigated for many different types of cancers.

Erbitux has been shown to improve the response rates in patients with advanced colorectal cancer when it is added to irinotecan therapy, as compared with irinotecan alone.

Erbitux and other monoclonal antibodies have a major advantage over standard chemotherapy agents: They produce fewer side effects, since only cancer cells are targeted. Even so, side effects can be seen and include diarrhea and an acne-like rash.

NEW CHEMOTHERAPY AGENTS

Some of the drugs on the horizon are newer forms of chemotherapy.

Raltitrexed (Tomudex)

Raltitrexed, an antimetabolite, is an intravenous agent that tricks cancer cells into thinking that it is a nutrient. Consequently, the cells take in the drug, their DNA is damaged, and the cells cannot divide. This drug is currently approved in Europe, but not in the United States.

UFT (Ftorafur and Uracil)

This combination of chemotherapy agents stops cells from manufacturing DNA and RNA, thereby halting the growth of cancer cells. Ftorafur is an antimetabolite that converts to 5-fluorouracil in the body; uracil is an amino acid (protein fragment) that enhances the effect of 5-fluorouracil. Together, these agents are used to treat colon cancer, as well as several other types of cancer, and are currently being tested in clinical trials. An advantage of UFT is that it can be taken as a pill, one hour before or after meals. This combination drug is approved in Japan, but not in the United States.

UFT (Uracil/Ftorafur) Plus Leucovorin (Orzel)

This combination, if approved, will offer another oral therapy for the treatment of advanced colorectal cancer. In clinical trials, it has been shown to shrink tumors and prolong survival as effectively as intravenous 5-fluorouracil and leucovorin, but with fewer side effects.

CANCER VACCINES

Cancer vaccines are designed to bolster the body's immune system. These vaccines show promise in the fight against cancer, and a number are now under investigation. Specifically, vaccines are designed to help your body's own immune system recognize and destroy precancerous and cancerous cells to fight cancer. Some vaccines are produced using a patient's own tumor cells, which are harvested during surgery, or by using abnormal proteins that are common to all cancer cells. These vaccines work by triggering the body's own immune system to attack tumor cells as if they were germs.

TYPES OF RADIATION THERAPY

Let me start by saying that radiation therapy is used primarily for rectal cancer, not colon cancer. Radiation therapy destroys cancer cells in two ways—by killing them directly and by preventing any surviving cells from growing and dividing. When treated with radiation, you must lie motionlessly on a flat table while the radiation dose is delivered over several minutes. You will be alone in the room but monitored by a radiologist on a television screen. Rest assured that you won't be glowing or radioactive after your treatment. Your doctor and radiologist determine the radiation dose and number of treatments based on the stage and location of the tumor, your health, and overall treatment goals.

The most widely used form of radiation is external beam radiation, in which short bursts of intense radiation, guided by a computer-driven machine, bombard and destroy cancer cells in the rectum. External beam radiation is given over a period of four to six weeks, following surgery. Usually, you can take an hour or so each day off from work to have your treatment, which is done as an outpatient at a hospital, clinic, or radiology facility.

Another form of radiation therapy exists, called endocavitary radiation, which employs an X-ray tube attached to a scope and inserted through the anus. The radiologist looks through the scope to see inside the rectum. That way, he or she can target the radiation directly at the tumor. This relatively new radiation procedure is often used as a primary treatment for rectal cancer.

MANAGING THE SIDE EFFECTS OF CHEMOTHERAPY AND RADIATION THERAPY

Chemotherapy and radiation therapy kill off cancer cells, but at the same time they indiscriminately damage normal, healthy cells, too, causing troublesome side effects. The most susceptible cells are those that rapidly divide, such as the cells found in hair follicles or in the lining of your mouth and gastrointestinal tract.

Some of the major side effects of these treatments are diarrhea, nausea, vomiting, loss of appetite, mouth sores, a rash on your hands and feet, and hair loss. Because chemotherapy, in particular, can harm the blood-producing cells of your bone marrow, you may have low blood cell counts. Though rare, low blood cell counts can increase your risk of infection, bleeding, bruising, and fatigue.

The side effects of radiation therapy are caused by the radiation beam striking healthy tissues in the path of the targeted area and include diarrhea, frequent urination, a rash in the groin, and decreased blood counts.

It is difficult to predict how long your side effects may last. A side effect such as a rash can last for a few weeks, while other side effects such as fatigue may persist for a few months, or longer, depending on how your body recovers following treatment. These side effects are not necessarily signs that your cancer has returned, but rather common problems that most people recovering from colorectal cancer go through.

There is simply no rhyme, reason, or normal pattern to side effects, but for most people, they get better over time. You can, however, avoid and minimize side effects, using the strategies I've listed for you in table 10-1. Please be sure to read chapter 11 very carefully, because it provides important advice on how to use certain complementary therapies such as meditation and relaxation to help resolve and control side effects.

Table 10-1

Treating the Side Effects of Chemotherapy and Radiation Therapy

Side Effect	Why It Occurs	Strategy
Diarrhea	This side effect is caused by the action of chemotherapy on the fast-dividing cells of your intestines.	• Drink lots of noncarbonated fluids to prevent dehydration and the loss of minerals and electrolytes. The best fluids are sports drinks such as Gatorade. • Avoid milk and dairy products. • Avoid diarrhea-producing substances such as alcohol, caffeine, sweets, and greasy or spicy foods. • Avoid high-fiber foods, which can promote diarrhea. • Eat small amounts of food throughout the day. These foods should include potassium-rich fruits and vegetables (bananas, oranges, and potatoes), unless your doctor has told you otherwise. Diarrhea can flush potassium from your body. • Ask your doctor about an over-the-counter medicine for diarrhea if it persists for more than 24 hours. • Call your doctor if you develop fever or chills.
Nausea and vomiting	Chemotherapy interferes with the normal function of cells lining your stomach and with certain cells in the brain that ordinarily control nausea. Radiation directed at the abdomen can also cause these side effects.	• Ask your doctor about medications that control nausea. • Eat several small meals throughout the day to avoid becoming full. • Eat slowly and chew your foods well. • Eat dry foods such as toast or crackers. • Drink small amounts of ginger ale or cola. • Stick to bland foods and avoid strong, spicy foods. • Avoid aromas that make you feel nauseous. • Breathe deeply when you feel nauseous and practice relaxation techniques.
Loss of appetite and change in taste	Depression or fatigue—both side effects of treatment—can make you lose your appetite. So can nausea and vomiting.	• Eat more frequently, but have smaller meals. • Sip nutritional beverages such as Boost or Ensure to make sure you take in nutrients. • Experiment with flavors to see what tastes best to you.
Mouth sores	Chemotherapy drugs travel throughout the body, damaging not only cancer cells but healthy cells as well. Among the	• Ask your doctor about medications to treat sores. • Use ice pops during therapy. • Drink lots of water. • Avoid spicy foods. • Stick to soft foods.

Side Effect	Why It Occurs	Strategy
	cells most likely to be damaged are those in the mouth.	• Brush and floss your teeth properly, using a soft toothbrush. • Avoid mouthwashes that contain salt or alcohol.
Rashes	Radiation causes the skin in the beam's path to become dry and irritated, much like a sunburn.	• Ask your doctor about a medication that will relieve the rash and the itching it may cause. Do not use lotions, creams, oils, or other remedies unless approved by your doctor. • Avoid scratching the rash to prevent infection. • Use mild soap and lukewarm water; do not scrub. • Stay out of the sun, or wear protective clothing when outside.
Fatigue	Chemotherapy can compromise bone marrow, and results in the declining production of red blood cells. This may lead to anemia, a frequent cause of fatigue. Dehydration from diarrhea may also cause fatigue. The overall effect of surgery, chemotherapy, and radiation on the body naturally causes fatigue.	• Engage in light exercise (such as walking). This may actually improve your fatigue, but don't overdo it. • Rest when you need to. • Maintain good nutrition. • Get help from friends to assist with activities such as child care, errands, housework, or driving.
Low blood counts (red cells and platelets)	Chemotherapy can damage the actively dividing cells in the bone marrow.	• Ask your doctor about an injection (procrit) that can increase your red cell counts. • Note any increased paleness to your lips, mouth, or skin tone. This is a sign of low red cells (medically known as anemia). • Note any unexpected bruises on your body and notify your doctor immediately. This is a sign that your platelets are too low. • Make sure your doctor monitors your blood counts with periodic blood tests.
Infections	A low white blood cell count leads to a weakening of your immune system.	• Watch for signs of infection (a fever higher than 100 degrees F, chills, sweats, coughing, pain with urination, and pain or redness around cuts or sores). If you feel an infection is coming on, notify your doctor right away. • Stay away from people who have diseases you can catch. This usually includes upper respiratory infections. • Practice good hygiene: Wash your hands frequently throughout the day and clean your rectal area thoroughly after each bowel movement. • Clean and treat cuts immediately. • Wear gloves when cleaning up after children and pets. • Use an electric shaver instead of a razor to prevent accidentally cutting your skin.

Side Effect	Why It Occurs	Strategy
Hair loss	Chemotherapy damages the fast-dividing cells of hair follicles.	• Use mild shampoos, soft hairbrushes, and low heat on your hair dryer. • Ask your oncologist if you can have your hair dyed or permed. • Have your hair cut short to make it look thicker and fuller. • Consider getting a wig if you have suffered hair loss. • Protect your scalp from the sun.

Dealing with Hair Loss

If your oncologist tells you that the drugs you're taking will cause hair loss (a condition known medically as alopecia), there is nothing you can do to prevent it. Here are some ways to make the experience more manageable:

▪ **If you are a woman:** Seeing your hair get thin and fall out is very depressing. So before you start chemotherapy, get a wig—a really beautiful one, in which you can still look great even without your own natural hair. I have seen many women look better than ever with the incredible wigs available today.

▪ **If you are a man:** Fortunately, baldness is more socially acceptable in men than in women. If you want the look of "hair" investigate toupees or wigs for men.

The good news for both men and women is that your hair will eventually regrow, although sometimes the quality of the new hair is different. For some people, that might not be such a bad thing.

SHOULD YOU PARTICIPATE IN A CLINICAL TRIAL?

There is an approach to treating colorectal cancer that may improve thousands of lives each year. Yet many doctors don't discuss it as an option. What is it? Participation in a clinical trial.

Clinical trials offer any early opportunity to try experimental drugs and treatments that have not yet been approved by the U.S. Food and Drug Administration (FDA). Scientists and researchers conduct trials only when they have reason to believe that the experimental treatment might be superior to standard treatment.

You may think that participating in a clinical trial makes you a guinea pig. It is true that there are known and unknown risks associated with a clinical trial. There are also potential benefits that could prolong or improve your life. Clinical trials are excellent for determining the safety and effectiveness of new drugs to treat, or even prevent, disease. Case in point: In the last three years, two new drugs have been approved for colon cancer; both were in clinical trials prior to approval. Therefore, the patients enrolled in those trials had access to these new drugs one to five years before other patients even heard about them. In a disease that does not wait, getting an early jump with a potentially better therapy may have substantial long-term benefits.

Many patients are concerned about getting a placebo (dummy pill). While many scientific studies do assign volunteers to a placebo group or to a treatment group, cancer studies usually do not. In clinical trials for cancer drugs not yet approved by the Food and Drug Administration, some people are assigned to the group receiving the most effective standard treatment, and others are assigned to a group getting the new experimental treatment. A computer randomly assigns you to each group, and you may not know which drug regimen you're taking.

Clinical trials must be conducted in three phases before they are eligible to win FDA approval. The purpose of a Phase I study is to determine the best way to administer the treatment and how much of it can be safely given to patients. Prior to Phase I trials, the treatment has been exhaustively studied in animals.

The goal of Phase II trials is to study the effectiveness of the treatment after its safety has been evaluated in Phase I. Doctors closely monitor patients for evidence of an anticancer effect by carefully measuring cancer sites that were present at the beginning of the trial. Side effects are closely watched, recorded, and assessed.

Phase III clinical trials involve thousands of people from across the nation. A control group of patients receives the standard treatment, while another group receives the experimental treatment. That way, doctors and researchers can compare the effect of both treatments to determine whether the new treatment enhances survival and quality of life. Side effects are closely monitored in this phase as well. A trial will be discontinued if side effects are too severe.

No matter what stage your cancer is in, you have the option of volunteering for a clinical trial, although it is an especially attractive option if you are undergoing palliative care. Here are important steps to take if you are interested in participating.

Explore Your Options

For a comprehensive list of ongoing cancer trials, you can check any number of resources. A good place to start is the National Cancer Institute (NCI) Web site at www.nci.nih.gov; or you can call the institute's cancer information service at 1-800-4-CANCER. Another helpful Web site is www.clinicaltrials.gov, a service of the National Institutes of Health (NIH), or call the NIH Clinical Center Patient Recruitment Office at 1-800-411-1222. The Jay Monahan Center for Gastrointestinal Health, which I direct, is currently compiling an exhaustive list of clinical trials. You can access this Web site at www.monahancenter.com.

Check with Your Insurance Company

The organizations and pharmaceutical companies that sponsor clinical trials pay for the cost of the therapy you receive. But there may be other costs that they don't pay for, including certain tests and drugs such as antinausea medications. Contact your health insurance company to verify whether your plan covers extra costs involved in participating in a clinical trial. If not, check with the study coordinator to see if the study will pay for additional blood tests, procedures, or medications.

Give Informed Consent

The doctors and medical personnel involved in the study will thoroughly explain the clinical trial to you, including the benefits and risks, and will give you a form to read and sign. Be sure to read it carefully and review it with your physician. This informed consent document states that you understand the potential risks and that you are volunteering to participate. Incidentally, signing the form does not mean you have to stay in the study after you have enrolled in it. You can leave the study at any time, for any reason.

Ask Questions

Before you decide to participate in a clinical trial, get answers to these questions:

- *What is the purpose of the trial?*
- *What is the experimental treatment designed to do?*
- *Am I a good candidate for a clinical trial?*
- *In what phase is the testing?*
- *What are the short- and long-term risks, side effects, and benefits of participating?*
- *What kind of tests, treatments, or hospitalization does the trial involve?*
- *Will I be able to tell if the treatment is working? If so, how?*

Volunteering for a clinical trial may be one of the best choices you can make to help treat your cancer, and indeed your doctor may encourage it, particularly if you are not responding to standard treatments. Not only may a clinical trial help you directly, but it may also help many other people with colorectal cancer in the future.

THE BOTTOM LINE

Don't fear chemotherapy, radiation therapy, or other treatments for colorectal cancer. They work. Clinical trials and scientific research are exploding with new, exciting chemotherapeutic and targeted agents. Understanding treatments for colorectal cancer, their potential side effects, and what you can do to minimize them, will put you in control of your disease, and not vice versa.

Chapter 11

Complementary Therapies for Colorectal Cancer

Colorectal cancer's current treatments—surgery, chemotherapy, and radiation therapy—have worked wonders in saving lives and creating multitudes of survivors. But anyone who has undergone these mainstream medical regimens, or witnessed their effects, knows firsthand that these treatments can be difficult.

The distress brought on by pain and other treatment-related side effects causes people to miss medical appointments, stop taking medications, and discontinue chemo- or radiation therapy altogether, compromising the effectiveness of treatment. Further, the discomfort and desperation that cancer brings can drive many people to seek out alternative treatments to a cancer cure, even though many of these treatments are untested, unproven, and unsafe.

Conventional cancer treatments like surgery, chemotherapy, and radiation therapy may be difficult and uncomfortable, but they are the only scientifically proven methods for treating, and in many cases, curing, colorectal cancer. Alternative treatments used instead of conventional therapies, such as herbal remedies, radical cancer diets, and so forth have not been shown to cure colorectal cancer— nor any other cancer, for that matter. So to choose an unproven alternative strategy over an established standard treatment can be tantamount to choosing death over life.

But this doesn't mean that nonconventional therapies have no legitimate place in mainstream medicine. They do—as long as they are used as *complementary* therapies; that is, to support established standard treatments, not to replace them. Used wisely, complementary therapies can make colorectal cancer, its symptoms, and its treatment and side effects more tolerable—and possibly even bolster the immune system for better recovery and healing.

If you ask your doctor about therapies such as acupuncture, meditation, or guided imagery, you may get a baffled, wide-eyed look. Your doctor is more likely to refer you to another physician than to a massage therapist or natural healer. That's because doctors, as a general rule, know very little about complementary therapies; nor are physicians very accepting of the fact that many nontraditional therapies may complement what they do—and help the body help itself along the way.

Fortunately, this is beginning to change. Many credible medical organizations, including the National Institute of Health (NIH) and American Cancer Society, along with a growing legion of cancer specialists, note certain complementary therapies as potentially helpful, when used in conjunction with established medical treatments, for easing pain, relieving side effects, and improving overall quality of life. In the information that follows, I'll explain some of the more credible complementary treatments and how they work; then I'll follow up by talking about therapies you should avoid at all costs.

ACUPUNCTURE

What Is It?

Once frowned upon by mainstream medicine, the ancient Chinese healing art of acupuncture is fast gaining respectability worldwide. In 1996, the FDA removed the "experimental" label from acupuncture needles as medical devices. And in the following year, the NIH concluded that acupuncture is effective against nausea and some pain, plus encouraged more research into the treatment. Acupuncture is used primarily to relieve pain and is now considered a legitimate pain-control technique.

How Well Does It Work?

As for the scientific evidence, numerous studies show that acupuncture is a viable treatment for pain, nausea, and vomiting, all of which are directly relevant to cancer patients.

In acupuncture, a licensed acupuncturist or physician inserts thin needles at specific pressure points on the body that affect physical or mental discomfort. The needles are left in place for anywhere from a few minutes to half an hour, and the procedure is virtually painless. Some have described it as feeling like a mosquito bite, or making a tingling sensation at the site of the puncture.

Is It Safe?

When performed by a trained, experienced professional, acupuncture has few risks. There is a slight chance of infection or bleeding at the puncture site, however. If your white blood count or platelet count is low due to chemotherapy, then I'd advise against having acupuncture due to the risk of infection.

ACUPRESSURE

What Is It?

A number of my patients have tried acupressure, a needle-free form of acupuncture, to reduce their dependence on pain medication and to help ease muscular tension. Acupressure is the ancient Chinese art of applying tension to the body's pressure points (or acupoints) with the fingertips, usually to help relax muscles. It is used frequently to alleviate pain in the shoulders, neck, face, or jaw, or to get rid of tension headaches.

How Well Does It Work?

Pain specialists use acupressure as a complementary therapy, and it is considered a form of manual healing. When you have acupressure, a trained therapist presses on acupoints with his or her fingers, rather than using needles.

There have been a few scientific studies involving acupressure as a complementary therapy in cancer treatment. Mainly, it has been shown to decrease chemotherapy-related nausea and vomiting.

Is It Safe?

Acupressure is generally safe, but you should not have it if you are experiencing pain stemming from arthritis, a muscle injury, or other insult to a body part. If you hate needles, this complementary therapy may be just what the doctor ordered.

AROMATHERAPY

What Is It?

Aromatherapy, which is one of the oldest forms of healing, employs essential oils that have been extracted from leaves, flowers, resins, seeds, fruit, grasses, wood, and other plant parts to alter mood or improve health. To achieve the desired effect, the oils are diffused into the air, burned as incense to permeate the atmosphere with a pleasing fragrance, diluted in bathwater, or massaged into the skin. There are more than forty oils used in aromatherapy; some of the most popular are lavender, rosemary, eucalyptus, chamomile, jasmine, and peppermint.

How Well Does It Work?

As a complementary therapy in cancer care, aromatherapy is promoted as a way to relieve pain, depression, and stress, and to achieve a feeling of well-being. When something, or someone, smells good, our bodies respond positively to the aroma by releasing feel-good substances called endorphins that induce tranquility. Indeed, there are a number of credible studies that attest to the relaxing effects of aromatherapy. In one study, cancer hospice patients who were exposed to lavender aromatherapy showed a slight improvement in their vital signs, depression, and levels of well-being.

If you want to try aromatherapy, the easiest way to get started is to purchase a plug-in diffuser at a health food store or from a massage therapist. Simply place a couple of droplets on one of the cotton pads that comes with the diffuser, and plug the diffuser into a wall socket. Use aromatherapy if you want to ease depression and anxiety; however, it has not been found to be an effective pain reliever.

Is It Safe?

Aromatherapy has few risks; the oils, however, should never be taken internally, since many are poisonous. Nor should these oils be applied directly to the skin, where they can cause irritation.

BIOFEEDBACK

What Is It?

Biofeedback is a therapeutic strategy that gives you conscious control over involuntary bodily reactions such as temperature changes, heart rate, blood pressure, and muscle tension that are ordinarily controlled automatically by your body. Biofeedback employs a special machine that, through electrodes attached to your skin, monitors minute changes in your body's physiological reactions. While hooked up to the machine and guided by a biofeedback therapist, you simultaneously use visualization and relaxation to help consciously regulate these functions. As you relax, the machine provides instant feedback on how well you're controlling the various functions. The ultimate goal is to achieve the desired relaxation response, but without the use of the machine.

How Well Does It Work?

In medicine, biofeedback has been used most extensively in the field of gastroenterology, primarily for the treatment of fecal incontinence (loss of bowel control) and constipation. Research has demonstrated that biofeedback helps strengthen sphincter muscles and improve rectal sensations for better control of bowel movements, particularly after colon surgery. For the relief of chronic constipation, this therapy has proven valuable in helping sphincter muscles and pelvic muscles properly relax in order to produce a normal bowel movement.

After reviewing the body of research on biofeedback, the NIH found the technique to be moderately effective for relieving chronic pain and approved biofeedback pain therapy.

Is It Safe?

Biofeedback is considered a safe therapy. It does require the help of a trained and certified professional to operate the equipment and interpret the changes. There are battery-operated devices you can use at home, but these haven't proven very reliable.

GUIDED IMAGERY

What Is It?

Just think: You're wheeled into the operating room, calm and stress-free. Afterward, your pain isn't as bad as it might have been. And your hospital stay is a day shorter than average. What gives?

Chalk it up to a technique called guided imagery. It involves using your imagination to visualize a specific image or goal, then imagining that you achieve it. In one study of guided imagery, 130 colorectal surgery patients were split into two groups: One half listened to voice and music tapes twice a day, for three days prior to surgery and six days afterward; the other half did not, although all the patients received the same standard care. The tapes were geared toward helping patients reduce their anxiety levels and be less frightened of surgery. Following surgery, those who listened to tapes needed less pain medication and experienced fewer side effects from the operation. What's more, their bowel function returned to normal more rapidly, and they were discharged from the hospital a day earlier than the patients in the other group.

How Well Does It Work?

One of the better-studied forms of complementary therapy, guided imagery relaxes the mind and body, and in doing so changes your physiology and your psychology, possibly to cue your body's own healing response. More than forty-five studies have found that guided imagery works for managing stress, anxiety, and the side effects of surgery, chemo- and radiation therapy.

You can learn this technique by working with a trained therapist, or by listening to pre-recorded audiotapes produced by the therapist. When you've acquired enough skill and practice, you can do guided imagery on your own. If you need to relax and calm down, for example, you might imagine yourself on a beautiful beach, with the sun against your skin or the waves lapping at your feet. The key is to evoke as many senses as possible: Smell the sea air, feel the warmth of the sun, and hear the sounds of the waves. One popular exercise is to imagine your body fighting off cancer cells. For instance, you might picture your immune cells attacking cancer cells in the diseased portion of your colon. Or, when you are receiving chemotherapy, you can imagine the medication flowing through your bloodstream and destroying the cancer cells.

There's no scientific evidence that guided imagery can cure cancer, or any other disease, but at least one study has demonstrated that it may increase survival rates for people with cancer. By that token, guided imagery is certainly worth a try.

Is It Safe?

Absolutely, especially when performed under the guidance of a trained therapist and used in conjunction with established cancer treatments. In fact, once you learn the principles of guided imagery, you can use this technique as a means of dealing with everyday stress. It really works.

HUMOR THERAPY

What Is It?

Groucho Marx once said, "A clown is like an aspirin, only he works twice as fast." There's a lot of truth to that, especially when you consider that laughter is truly one of the best medicines—and a terrific stress reliever. Plus, it stimulates the release of special substances called endorphins in the brain that help control pain. For this and other health reasons, humor therapy is now widely used in hospitals across the country to help patients reduce stress, ease pain, encourage relaxation, promote health, and enhance quality of life.

How Well Does It Work?

Humor therapy involves two approaches—passive humor, in which you watch a comedy or read a joke book or the funny papers; and humor production, in which you learn to create humor or find the lighter side of a stressful situation.

A sense of humor can be one of your greatest allies in the battle against cancer. When patients have truly lost their ability to laugh or smile, I know that they are either severely depressed or losing the battle against cancer. Research into the medical benefits of humor therapy has found that its use helps control and reduce pain levels. What's more, laughter—an end product of humor—decreases levels of stress hormones in the body, leading to a stress-relieving effect. So if nothing seems funny to you right now, maybe it's a good time to rent a comedy video, go to a comedy club, or read a humorous book. If nothing still seems funny, discuss this with your doctor, because it might be a clue to an underlying depression.

Is It Safe?

As you might guess, there's absolutely no harm in using humor therapy. Of course, laughter can cause pressure on a fresh abdominal incision giving credibility to the saying "It only hurts when I laugh." But in all sincerity, I believe humor therapy is fun, beneficial, and probably best stated in another great saying: "He who laughs, lasts."

MASSAGE THERAPY

What Is It?

Massage therapy is a hands-on technique of rubbing, kneading, and working the muscles of the body in order to bring about relaxation. There's no question that massage is one of the best stress soothers around. It relaxes muscles that have tensed up due to mental strain and anxiety and allows more oxygen and nutrients to reach cells by improving circulation and blood flow. Plus, studies show that massage releases brain chemicals that improve mood.

Not all massages are alike, however. There are different types that address different types of problems. The Swedish massage, for example, is an excellent massage for stress because it relaxes tension. Deep muscle massage, which goes a little deeper, is also beneficial for relieving stress, too, since it releases tension from the body. Regardless of what type you have, a massage should be performed by a certified therapist.

How Well Does It Work?

Massage is a useful technique for cancer patients because of its stress-relieving benefits. In one study, cancer patients who underwent just thirty minutes of hands-on massage two nights in a row experienced less pain, reduced anxiety, and great relaxation. The researchers concluded that massage "is a beneficial nursing intervention that promotes relaxation and alleviates the perception of pain and anxiety in hospitalized cancer patients."

A study on the effects of massage on the immune systems of HIV-positive patients revealed that a month's worth of massage therapy increased significantly the number of "natural killer cells" in the patients' bodies. Natural killer cells are white blood cells containing grenadelike granules filled with lethal chemicals. When they encounter an invading agent such as a virus, these cells jump onto the invader, take aim, and release their chemicals. Based on these findings, it looks as though massage causes something good to happen at the level of cellular immunity, and as the researchers pointed out in this study, this benefit may have implications for cancer patients.

Is It Safe?

Generally, massage is safe, but if you have any muscle or skeletal problems you should tell the massage therapist so that the affected areas will be left out of the massage and not harmed.

MEDITATION

What Is It?

Originating in ancient India some three thousand years ago, meditation is one of several relaxation methods approved by the NIH for easing chronic pain and insomnia. No one yet knows whether it is effective in treating cancer, though it can certainly help improve quality of life if you have cancer. You can practice meditation on your own, or under the guidance of a trained therapist, psychiatrist, or other qualified health professional.

How Well Does It Work?

Meditation has been well studied for the past fifteen years. Research confirms that it reduces anxiety, stress, blood pressure, chronic pain, and sleeplessness. In addition, an NIH group uncovered evidence that regular meditation can help regulate cholesterol levels in the body, reduce substance abuse, increase longevity, and enhance quality of life.

Emptying your mind and relaxing your body are two of the main goals of meditation. These produce a decrease in blood pressure and a leveling off of stress hormones. Both effects diminish feelings of anxiety, and this can be of great value to cancer patients.

To meditate, find a quiet place, free from noise and distractions. Sit quietly with your eyes closed and try to achieve a feeling of peace. Concentrate on a pleasant idea or thought, while repeating a phrase, a Scripture verse, or something that is meaningful to you. If your mind wanders, return your attention to the pleasant image in your mind and keep repeating the phrase. Focus on your breathing as well. The point is to separate yourself mentally from the outside world and free yourself from intrusive, negative thoughts.

Is It Safe?

In rare, isolated cases, meditation has produced adverse mental symptoms, including anxiety, depression, and confusion, but these tend to occur in people who have preexisting mental disorders. Most experts concur that the positive benefits of meditation outweigh any potentially negatives.

MUSIC THERAPY

What Is It?

There is an incredibly simple method for reducing pain and chemotherapy-induced nausea and vomiting—something that many of us are already doing and loving: listening to music. Because of its soothing ability, music is often used to treat a variety of physical, emotional, and psychological symptoms in patients, and it is employed frequently in cancer treatment to ease side effects. Music therapy involves not only listening to the music of your choice, but also songwriting and musical performances.

How Well Does It Work?

Numerous clinical trials have verified the benefit of using music therapy in cancer care for relieving pain from cancer. Patients who opt to use music therapy often have to take less medication. Research has found that music therapy and antinausea drugs, when given to patients undergoing high-dose chemotherapy, greatly reduce the symptoms of nausea and vomiting. Other research has discovered that music therapy eases depression and anxiety in patients undergoing radiation therapy for cancer. We recently installed music in each procedure room at the NewYork-Presbyterian Hospital/Weill Cornell endoscopy suite to help reduce the fear and anxiety that develop before a procedure. There is no question in my mind—it works!

No one yet knows for sure how music therapy confers its healing benefits, but there are some theories. One holds that your muscles, including your heart muscle, learn to synchronize with the beat and rhythm of the music. Another theory hints that music distracts your mind and keeps you from focusing on your pain and stress.

Certified music therapists working in hospitals, cancer centers, hospices, and other health care settings design music sessions for individuals or groups, based on personal musical needs and tastes. But you can certainly do music therapy on your own. Just turn on your stereo, put on your headphones or whatever, and listen to your favorite soothing music in a relaxed setting. It's a great way to harmonize your mind, body, and spirit.

If there's a cancer treatment, medical test, or surgery in your future, plug into music therapy to defuse moments of anxiety and to feel calmer. Many surgery centers, in fact, now give their patients a portable CD player with headphones and music to listen to prior to their operation. If your doctor doesn't do this, tell him that you're bringing your CD or tape player, headphones, and music in to listen to before and after your procedure. Usually, your doctor and other health care staff will be happy to accommodate you.

Is It Safe?

Music therapy is certainly a wonderful and effective complement to cancer treatment, with absolutely no downside.

PRAYER

What Is It?

More than ever, prayer has been in the spotlight as a not-to-be-ignored phenomenon in health and healing. And as doctors, we know that religion and faith are very important to many of our patients dealing with cancer and other diseases. The spiritual dimension of people's lives helps them cope with illness, lessens stress and anxiety, promotes a positive outlook, and strengthens their will to live. There is also a documented scientific link between faith and mental health. People who are religious or come from a religious family have a lower risk of suicide, mental illness, drug abuse, alcoholism, and depression.

Prayer takes many forms and is practiced in numerous ways. Prayer can be silent or spoken out loud, done alone or in groups. It may involve prayer on your own behalf, or prayer for someone else (intercessory prayer). Many hospitals and medical institutions include prayer as an important part of healing and have chaplains, ministers, rabbis, and other clergy to help with patients' spiritual needs.

How Well Does It Work?

Scientific explorations of prayer have been mixed, but many show that prayer and religion have a positive impact on physical and mental health. Even so, the whole area of prayer and healing is embroiled in controversy, so rather than jumping into the debate, let me say that for people of faith, prayer, as well as involvement in a spiritual community, does make them feel better and stronger. With all the suffering cancer can bring, prayer helps people take stock of their lives by addressing their hopes and fears and this attitude strengthens and sustains them in their battle against cancer.

Is It Safe?

There are certainly no health risks associated with prayer, but patient consent is important before pursuing any activity, including prayer, that may influence health. Of course, there are people who do not believe in prayer or spiritual healing and may object to being prayed for. Further, relying on prayer alone and shunning medical treatments can result in a serious and potentially life-threatening outcome.

PROGRESSIVE MUSCLE RELAXATION

What Is It?

Progressive muscle relaxation is another form of relaxation therapy designed to encourage calm, but one that stands out among others because it has been so extensively researched. Developed in the 1930s, progressive muscle relaxation is a method in which you learn to contract and relax various muscles in your body. This brings about relaxation and a general sense of well-being. Progressive muscle relaxation is now widely used as complementary therapy to treat a number of medical conditions.

How Well Does It Work?

There is plenty of scientific evidence showing that progressive muscle relaxation is effective for treating insomnia, headaches, and mental stress. A meta-analysis (statistical study) revealed that this technique improved the ability of cancer patients to withstand chemotherapy. Another study found that progressive muscle relaxation, when employed with guided imagery (an often used combination), reduced mental stress in cancer patients.

As with meditation and guided imagery, progressive muscle relaxation is something you can learn to do under the guidance of a qualified therapist, or on your own through practice, by alternately tensing and relaxing your muscles, one muscle group at a time, in sequence.

Is It Safe?

Like most forms of relaxation therapy, progressive muscle therapy has no side effects and is certainly worth a try, particularly if you're suffering from anxiety and stress.

T'AI CHI

What Is It?

This ancient Chinese form of martial arts is a healing system that uses movement, meditation, and breathing to enhance health and well-being. When practicing t'ai chi, you concentrate on natural motions, strength building, and relaxation to clear your mind. You begin by learning a series of gentle, nonimpact exercises called forms. The forms contain between twenty and a hundred moves that require twenty minutes to complete. The names of the forms come from nature; for example, *wave hands like clouds*. While doing these exercises, you should focus on your breathing and technique.

How Well Does It Work?

Much research has examined the benefits of t'ai chi, with impressive findings. T'ai chi improves posture, balance, flexibility, muscle tone, and strength. It also has been found to reduce heart rate and blood pressure. Evidence from other research indicates that t'ai chi reduces amounts of stress hormones in the body, suggesting that it can diminish tension, anxiety, and mood disturbances. That being so, t'ai chi certainly is beneficial as a complementary therapy to conventional cancer care.

Is It Safe?

T'ai chi is relatively safe. If you have severe balance problems, arthritis, or other physical limitations, get your doctor's okay before participating in t'ai chi, because it involves a lot of moves that require good balance.

YOGA

What Is It?

Practiced for more than five thousand years, yoga is a form of non-aerobic exercise that incorporates an assortment of postures, or asanas, coupled with deep breathing. It is often used to complement cancer treatment because it stimulates relaxation, eases muscular tension, and fosters positive mental health.

How Well Does It Work?

A growing number of people with cancer are using yoga to help them deal with the physical and emotional aspects of the disease. Yoga stretches your muscles, makes you feel more energized, and enhances your flexibility. Many hospitals and clinics are now offering yoga classes as part of their complementary therapy programs.

The NIH reports that there is evidence that yoga complements conventional cancer treatments by relieving symptoms associated with cancer, such as pain and stress. Indeed, studies show that yoga does reduce stress and produce feelings of relaxation and well-being.

Is It Safe?

Some yoga postures are difficult to do and may be hard on your body. Make sure you consult your doctor before trying yoga. There's a low-impact form of yoga called Kripalu that is recommended for cancer patients because it is not strenuous and places minimal stress on your joints. Look for a class, or a videotape you can use at home, that practices this form of yoga.

PSYCHOTHERAPY

I list psychotherapy at the end of this chapter not because it is a "holistic" measure but because it is a true complementary therapy in the sense that it adds significantly to your ability to cope with life's stressors. And let me remind you that cancer is certainly one of them. Because depression and anxiety can hurt your quality of life, and to some extent your body's healing response, it is a wise decision to pursue psychotherapy while dealing with cancer.

What Is It?

Psychotherapy involves meeting with a qualified mental health therapist to learn positive ways to cope with cancer, understand the reasons for your particular defense mechanisms and behaviors, as well as to tap into your inner strength in order to live more fully.

How Well Does It Work?

There are many different kinds of therapy; four of the best choices for cancer patients are cognitive-behavioral therapy, supportive psychotherapy, pain management counseling, and support groups.

• **Cognitive-behavioral therapy** is based on the premise that your troublesome physical and mental symptoms are a consequence of negative and irrational thoughts and feelings. With cognitive-behavioral therapy, you learn how to slip out of self-defeating thought patterns and think more positively and realistically about the world around you. This form of therapy employs a number of strategies that I've discussed here, including progressive muscle relaxation and guided imagery, to help change your thoughts and behavior in a positive manner. Cognitive-behavioral strategies have been extensively used, with great success, to help alleviate chemotherapy-related nausea and vomiting. When relaxation strategies are used as part of the therapy, pain is better controlled, too.

• **Supportive psychotherapy** employs several different formats, including individual, family, couples, and group therapy. Its goal is to help you manage your limitations while continuing to live your life with meaning and purpose. Your therapist helps you set goals and design strategies for dealing with stress and for managing pain. You'll be encouraged to talk about your feelings, get them out in the open, and explore practical issues that are affecting your adjustment to cancer. Research into the benefit of supportive therapy has found that cancer patients who use this therapeutic approach have more energy, feel less tense and depressed, and experience a decrease in their pain levels.

• **Pain management counseling** empowers patients to actively participate in pain control strategies. This is critical, because pain stresses the immune system and interferes with the body's healing response. With this approach, a counselor provides education on how you can assess your pain, control it, and use your pain medications effectively, along with nondrug approaches to pain management. You might be asked, for example, to keep a daily pain diary or log that documents the time and date of a pain experience, its severity, and what you did to alleviate it. The idea behind pain management counseling is that the more personal control you have over your pain, the more you can do to prevent pain as a side effect. Indeed, studies have found that educating patients about pain control increases compliance with pain medication, decreases the fear of addiction, lessens pain intensity and severity, and reduces anxiety.

• **Support groups** are composed of cancer patients without professional leaders. They are run by patients for patients. People with colorectal cancer get to share their personal experiences and strategies for coping. You can hear, firsthand, what others with cancer have gone through. By joining a support group, you will be surrounded by people who understand exactly how you are feeling. For more information concerning support groups see page 220, "Seek and Embrace Support."

Is It Safe?

In whatever form it takes, psychotherapy is an excellent complement to conventional cancer treatment. It can help you control pain, probe your depression and anxiety, give you constructive guidelines for resolving the crucial issues you're facing. Other than support groups, psychotherapy must be conducted by a certified mental health professional.

ALTERNATIVE AND COMPLEMENTARY THERAPIES TO AVOID

While there are many complementary therapies that work against cancer in beneficial ways, there are a lot of therapies that are bogus, completely useless, unproven, and perhaps even harmful. I've listed a number of them for you in table 11-1.

If you are considering a complementary therapy, the American Cancer Society advises that you use the following checklist, a grading scale of sorts, to evaluate whether the treatment makes sense or nonsense.

- Is the treatment based on an unproven or disproved theory? In other words, is there any credible scientific data available to support its use and back its claims?
- Does the treatment promise a cure for cancer? (A yes answer here is a showstopper.)
- Do the promoters of the treatment tell you not to use conventional medicine?
- Is the drug or treatment a "secret" that only certain providers or manufacturers can give?
- Does the therapy require you to travel to another country for the "cure"?
- Do the promoters of the therapy attack mainstream medicine and its physicians?

If you can answer yes to even one of these questions, you're being duped by the promoters and providers of the treatment. There are many charlatans who only want your money and care nothing about your cancer. Don't waste your time, money, energy, or health chasing after something that could jeopardize you, physically and mentally.

It is enticing to hear about an alternative therapy that "cures" cancer. Trust me, I know this lesson all too well, because my own mother was diagnosed with ovarian cancer. You want so much to believe that there is something out there you can latch on to that will cure you, or someone you love, just like in the movies. Reality, though, can be so difficult to accept, and the promise of a cure so seductive.

But like anything else, if it sounds too good to be true, then it's not true. Don't let yourself fall into this trap! Hope is important, but false hope can be very harmful.

Let me encourage you to talk to your physician and other health care providers about any decisions you make to pursue complementary therapies. The fact that many doctors are unfamiliar with the use, risks, and potential benefits of these treatments should not dissuade you from a frank, open discussion, especially if you reassure your doctor that a complementary therapy will not interfere with the medical treatment he or she has prescribed. Who knows? You might even teach your doctor a thing or two.

Table 11-1

Don't Use These Unproven and Dangerous Therapies

Therapy	Unproven Claims	What's Involved	Risks/Fallacies
Alternative cancer diets	Claim to prevent or cure cancer.	These diets typically emphasize avoiding meat, and many are strictly vegetarian.	Although there are positive aspects to some cancer diets, many exclude vital nutrients; no diet has been shown to cure cancer.
Bioelectromagnetics	Promoted as a way to heal damaged tissues, including cancer.	Uses magnetic fields to penetrate the body and supposedly promote healing .	No scientific studies exist to support the claims of bioelectromagnetics.
Cancell	A product that claims to return cancer cells to their "primitive state" so that they can be digested and turned inert.	Taken as a supplement.	The product contains common chemicals, including nitric acid, sodium sulfite, and potassium hydroxide, which provide no therapeutic benefit and may be toxic.

Therapy	Unproven Claims	What's Involved	Risks/Fallacies
Chinese herbal medicine	Claims to prevent a host of health problems including cancer.	Involves various herbs used medicinally.	May cause serious injury to the gastrointestinal tract, including liver toxicity.
Coffee enemas	Promoted as part of several controversial cancer regimens.	Enemas containing coffee are given to flush out the rectum in the belief that this will relieve pain, nausea, and other symptoms.	Electrolyte depletion; irritation of tissues.
Colon therapy (also called detoxification therapy)	Cleansing or detoxifying the colon supposedly increases the efficiency of the body's natural healing abilities; promoted as a treatment for illness.	Plastic tubes are inserted through the rectum and into the colon. A pump shoots water (up to 20 gallons) containing herbs and enzymes into the colon. The abdomen is massaged to facilitate removal of waste from the colon out of the body through another tube, The procedure is repeated several times; a session lasts 45 to 60 minutes.	Infection and death from contaminated equipment; death from electrolyte depletion; perforation of colon wall. There is no "toxic waste" that resides in the colon.
Essiac	Promoted as an alternative treatment for cancer.	Taken as a supplement, which contains four herbs: burdock, turkey rhubarb, sorrel, and slippery elm.	Researchers at the National Cancer Institute (NCI) and elsewhere have not found this herbal combination to have any anticancer effect. It is illegal in Canada.
Megavitamin therapy	Promoted as a cancer cure.	Massive dosages of vitamin C and other antioxidants are taken as an anticancer regimen.	Large doses of vitamin C can protect tumors from chemotherapy and radiation.
Shark cartilage	Promoted as a cancer cure, based on the notion that sharks don't get cancer—an idea that has since been refuted by marine biologists.	Shark cartilage is available in supplement form; a protein within the cartilage is supposed to inhibit antiogenesis, the growth of blood vessels that provide sustenance to tumors.	There are no apparent side effects from taking these supplements, unless you consider a waste of your money a side effect.

Therapy	Unproven Claims	What's Involved	Risks/Fallacies
		The molecules of this protein in the supplements, however, are too large for absorption into the bloodstream.	

Adapted from: Cassileth, B.R. 1999. Evaluating complementary and alternative therapies for cancer patients. CA:*A Cancer Journal for Clinicians* 49:362–375; and Ernst, E. 2001. A primer of complementary and alternative medicine commonly used by cancer patients. *Medical Journal of Australia* 174: 88–92.

What is involved in follow-up care?

Regular follow-up care is vital, because your doctor can monitor your progress and make sure that the cancer has not returned (recurrence), or spread to other parts of your body (metastasized). Normally, you'll continue to be evaluated and treated by the same doctor who provided your cancer treatment, usually your oncologist, and you'll need to see him or her at specific intervals for up to five years. (For other medical care, continue to see your primary care doctor.)

Once you're discharged from the hospital, you'll be scheduled for follow-up appointments every three to four months for the first two years after treatment.

At each follow-up visit, your doctor will review your medical history, discuss any unusual symptoms you're experiencing, perform a thorough physical examination, and run some follow-up tests.

These tests may include a CEA blood test, chest X rays, and sometimes a CT scan, an MRI, or ultrasound. A colonoscopy will often be recommended at six months to one year after surgery. Many doctors now have their patients undergo a PET scan for the early detection of recurrent colorectal cancer.

In addition to the follow-up tests your doctor orders, you should definitely have a colonoscopy within the first three years following your cancer diagnosis. If no disease is detected, your doctor will advise that colonoscopies every three to five years should be a part of your ongoing follow-up. It bears repeating: Colorectal cancer testing is the best way to catch a recurrence or new cancer early. Don't let anxiety or a busy schedule interfere with doing something that could keep you well.

After five years, if all goes well, and there have been no signs of a recurrence, you'll need to see your oncologist only once a year. Remember that the goal of follow-up is to detect the possible recurrence of cancer. If your cancer has not returned, follow-ups every three to five years, especially to detect new polyps, are advisable for the rest of your life.

During your follow-up visits, bring a friend or family member with you—someone who can remember and help you understand everything your doctor said. Consider taking notes in order to have

Chapter 12

Life After Colorectal Cancer

With your cancer treatment behind you, it is understandable, and perfectly normal, for you to be concerned about what lies ahead. Maybe you're wondering about how long it will take to start feeling like your old self again. Maybe in the back of your mind, you're worried about whether your cancer will return. Maybe you want to know what you can do to prevent it from coming back, or how to cope with any lingering effects of treatment.

Concerns, worries, and fears like these can be overwhelming, tumbling down with all the force of an avalanche. I know because these are the same feelings my own patients have. As I do with them, I will give you information in this chapter that will help you learn about what to expect from this point forward, what you can do about your health and wellness, and what actions you can take in order to move on with your life.

One by one, I'll answer for you the questions I know are on your mind. When you understand what life is like after cancer, you'll be able to regain the sense of control you felt you lost during treatment and put your life back in order. And you'll feel less fearful about the future. Feeling in control and focusing on wellness will enhance your recovery, help you heal, and make your life feel whole once again.

Part IV

LIVING WELL AFTER COLORECTAL CANCER

a record of your conversations with your doctor. It is also a good idea to bring a list of symptoms or questions with you, so you can make productive use of your appointment.

What is the role of my primary care physician?

He or she should stay up to date on your earlier cancer treatment and your cancer-related medical history, in the event that you happen to develop suspicious medical problems after your active cancer treatment has ended and you are no longer seeing your oncologist on a regular basis. Your primary care doctor should keep in your medical file copies of the following information: details of all your cancer treatments; medications you took; lab reports; pathology reports; imaging and X-ray reports; any problems you encountered during treatment; and information on complementary care you received. Make sure your doctor has these records.

If my colon or rectal cancer returns, how will I know?

Even if your colorectal cancer is in remission, there is, unfortunately, the chance that it can come back. Most relapses occur within five years of initial diagnosis and treatment, although the highest rate of return is within eighteen months of treating the first cancer. Colorectal cancer can recur in other organs of the body, including the liver, lining of the abdomen, and lungs but rarely in the brain, spine, and bones. In addition, colorectal cancer can recur at the point where the colon was removed and rejoined (the anastamosis) or, uncommonly, in a different place in the colon.

The odds of a recurrence are related to the stage at which your cancer was first detected. For example, if your cancer was caught early and confined to your colon wall, then a recurrence is much less likely than if your cancer had spread to your lymph nodes at the time of your diagnosis. Recurrence, however, is not necessarily a death sentence. It can be treated with surgery, chemotherapy, radiation therapy, or a combination of these, just as your original cancer was treated.

Do not be afraid to ask your doctor about the recurrence rate and long-term survival rates for your particular situation. Your doctor will answer that question using statistical averages. You should treat those statistics only as pieces of information to help you and your family plan and take control of your health and recovery following your treatment. Remember that statistics do not take into account the newer surgical techniques and advances in chemotherapy. And they don't predict what will happen to you as an individual. So listen to the numbers but don't depend on them—and never, ever give up hope.

Because you'll see your doctors only at certain intervals, you must take responsibility for your health the rest of the time. Listen to what your body is telling you and how you feel, and be alert to any unusual changes in your bowel habits and overall health, including your energy level and weight loss or gain. Note any pain that is troubling you. Bring these symptoms to the attention of your doctor, no matter how trivial you may think they are. Let your doctor decide what's important and what's not.

In the sidebar, I've listed a number of symptoms that could point to a potential problem with the healing of your colon or a recurrence of colon or rectal cancer. Of course, if you experience any of these symptoms, it is important that your doctor give you a complete checkup, with the appropriate battery of tests.

What to Watch For

- Fever
- Persistent constipation that does not respond to laxatives.
- Persistent diarrhea.
- Chronic abdominal pain, bloating, or fullness.
- Persistent nausea or vomiting.
- Change in stool quality.
- Change in stool color.
- Rectal bleeding (dark or bright red blood).

- Constant urge to have a bowel movement, even though you have just had one.

- Excess mucus secretions with bowel movements.

- Poor appetite.

- Fatigue or dizziness.

- Unexplained weight loss.

- Persistent cough.

- Frequent headaches.

- Yellowing of eyes or skin (jaundice).

What lifestyle changes should I make?

After being treated for colorectal cancer, so many of my patients tell me that they've had a loud wake-up call. They start taking a hard look at themselves, how they've been living, and what they need to do to take better care of themselves for the future. Often, cancer survivors have a new appreciation of life and can better prioritize what is important and what is not. Through this wake-up call, they find what is "good" about having cancer, even though it seemed like the worst of times, and this new awareness helps them focus on the positive aspects of their lives and make changes in order to stay as healthy as possible. What follows is an action plan, a road map, to help you make similar changes—in the way you eat and exercise, as well as in your day-to-day habits.

EAT NUTRITIOUSLY AFTER YOUR CANCER TREATMENT

Healthy eating can't take the place of medical therapies following surgery and other treatments, but it will certainly enhance those therapies. The diet I outlined for you in chapter 5 for prevention is exactly the same approach you should take to stay healthy following your active cancer treatment. It's a diet that's low in saturated and trans fats, high in fiber, low in sugar and processed foods, low in red meat, and high in fruits, vegetables, and whole grains.

Keeping tabs on your daily caloric intake is important, since eating too much food stresses the digestive system. There is some evidence showing that a high level of calories in your diet, regardless of whether the source is fat, carbohydrate, or protein, may favor the development of cancer. In other words, the more food that passes through your colon, the higher your risk. Most people should eat no more than two thousand calories a day—an amount that helps keep pounds from piling on, especially if you stay active and exercise regularly. This is good advice for anyone who wants to stay healthy.

SUPPLEMENT YOUR DIET

One supplement that more doctors should be prescribing for women is calcium. Some clinical trials show that calcium can help keep polyps from growing back and can increase survival rates among patients who have been treated for colorectal cancer. The Calcium Polyp Prevention Study, for example, studied the effect of calcium on colon cancer, using 930 people with a history of the disease. The participants took 1,200 milligrams of calcium, or a placebo, for four years. When compared to the placebo group, the calcium supplementers had a 15 percent reduction in the recurrence of polyps, and when polyps did return, they were fewer in number. If your doctor agrees that calcium supplementation is worth a try, take at least 1,200 milligrams a day, the amount used in most of the clinical trials (see page 97). (As a reminder, I don't recommend calcium supplementation to men, because of the possible elevated risk of prostate cancer.)

It also makes sense to supplement with folic acid when not undergoing cancer treatment. (400 micrograms—the amount found in most multivitamin/mineral supplements). Folic acid has been shown in numerous studies to decrease the risk of cancer (see page 94). Vitamin D, up to 800 IUs daily, is also a good idea if you are not getting enough in your diet or from exposure to sunlight (see page 101).

TAKE ASPIRIN

More and more doctors across the country, myself included, are advising high-risk patients to take an aspirin a day to decrease the risk of colorectal cancer. Some very convincing studies indicate that aspirin is a potential shield against colon cancer. Remember, though, aspirin can be associated with serious side effects, including life-threatening gastrointestinal bleeding. So please do not start taking aspirin until you have discussed the risks and benefits with your doctor.

DRINK ENOUGH WATER

Drinking enough water each day (at least eight glasses of pure water) is vital to the health of your colon—and indeed to your entire digestive system. Water helps separate stool from the mucous lining of your colon, assists in stimulating the muscular movement of your intestines, and keeps material flowing through your system at a healthy rate. If you're chronically low on water (dehydrated), this can lead to hard bowel movements, constipation, diverticulitis, and hemorrhoids.

AVOID OR LIMIT ALCOHOL

If you have been treated for colorectal cancer, my recommendation is to minimize alcohol intake, since it is a risk factor for this disease and other cancers such as esophageal cancer. In addition, alcohol is damaging to the liver, stomach, and intestine. So why play with fire? If you enjoy having a drink or two, switch to nonalcoholic beer or wine, or have carbonated water with a twist of lemon or lime.

EXERCISE DAILY

Because exercise is such a powerful means of staying healthy and energetic it is an important component of rehabilitation following cancer treatment. Physical activity helps regulate insulin, insulin-like growth factor, bile acid levels, and other potential cancer-triggering substances in your body. Exercise also increases the speed of intestinal movement, thereby reducing the contact between possible carcinogens in the feces and the lining of your colon.

There's more: Another benefit of regular exercise is that it strengthens your immune system, not only in healthy people, but also in patients who have had or are undergoing cancer treatments. This means that exercise may ultimately help cancer survivors live longer. There are emotional advantages, too: less anxiety and depression, improved mood, and stronger self-esteem.

Getting regular exercise is vital to your follow-up care. One of the easiest and best exercises is daily walking, performed for at least half an hour each day. Using treadmills, stair-climbing machines, and stationary bikes are other options that provide the same benefits. After your treatment and with your doctor's approval, start your exercise program slowly and build your activity over time.

STOP SMOKING

Because of some convincing scientific data, we believe that smoking and tobacco usage can increase the odds of developing colorectal cancer at the same site or at another site. Moreover, smoking is terrible for your overall health because it causes lung cancer, heart disease, and vascular disease. So one of the best things you can do for yourself is stop smoking. If you need help quitting, you can consult your doctor and enroll in a smoking cessation program.

KEEP YOUR OTHER REGULAR HEALTH CHECKUPS

To guard your overall health, don't forget about other recommended cancer prevention and screening exams. Although colorectal cancer has been the center of your life in the recent past, you must also keep up with other important cancer-screening tests. If you're a woman, have a yearly mammogram starting at age forty, along with an annual Pap smear. Men should get rectal prostate exams starting at age 40 and annual prostate-specific antigen (PSA) blood tests beginning at age fifty. High-risk men or African American men should start PSA testing at age forty.

Obviously, life after cancer is different physically, at least for a while. But it is also different emotionally. Your outlook, the way you think and feel, and indeed your very spirit may be radically affected. Just as you take care of your body, you need to take care of your emotions, because they play such a pivotal role in your healing—even your survival. Turn the page and explore with me the importance of harnessing the power of hope and finding positive meaning in your life.

Chapter 13

Healing from Within

Hope, meaning, and the belief in good things. These are the essential human components that inspire us, feed our soul, and sustain us emotionally and spiritually. We all recognize the importance of these qualities in our lives, but sometimes the pace of the day-to-day life can leave them somewhere in the background. From my work as a doctor, I know that nothing moves the important things to the forefront of life quicker than a diagnosis of cancer in yourself or someone you love. But these are the very things that can help you and your family get through the cancer experience.

If you, or someone you love has been diagnosed with cancer, maintaining a sense of hope and meaning in your life can help you to feel better emotionally and spiritually—and sometimes even physically. In keeping your eye on the positive, you can begin to give your spirit the nurturing it needs and heal from within.

THE MIND–BODY CONNECTION

Medically and psychologically, there is no denying the effect of extreme worry, stress, fear, and sadness on the body. Nowhere is this more true than the gastrointestinal system. Scientists have known for a long time that there is a direct connection between your brain and your gut. There are nerves entrenched in the lining of the esophagus, stomach, small intestine, and colon, and your brain communicates with these nerves. When faced with a stress-provoking event, for example, your brain sends messages to these nerves, and a physical response is registered in the form of butterflies in your stomach, cramping in your intestines, or some other form of gut-level discomfort. The colon, in particular, is very sensitive to stress and emotional turmoil. You've probably noticed this yourself when you've been under stress and your bowel habits change to diarrhea or constipation.

It is not just the gastrointestinal system that is hard hit, but also your immune system. Every negative thought or emotion you have can put a great deal of stress on your body's defenses.

This is not to say that we cause our own illness. We all know that even the most positive-thinking person can be struck with cancer. It is also not to say that feelings of sadness, anger, and fear are going to compromise your treatment or recovery. These feelings are normal, especially after a cancer diagnosis. But you can harness the power of a positive attitude—nurturing a sense of hope, meaning, and connectedness—to help foster an environment of ease and healing in your life. That's right. Your attitudes and your mood can exert a powerful effect on the state of your health.

Positive psychological traits such as hopefulness, self-reliance, self-empowerment, loving relationships, and faith—whether in your doctors, in your own power to heal, or in a higher power—can go a long way to enhancing the quality and possibly even the length of our lives. And, in some cases, these traits have been shown to influence long-term prognosis. A case in point: In a small but rather intriguing study conducted at the Ontario Cancer Institute a few years back, researchers studied twenty-two people with incurable forms of cancer—breast, colon, rectum, and pancreas—and discovered that those who made healing the top priority in their lives, who worked the hardest at changing their inner psychology, and who were the most open to doing so, lived at least three years longer than what oncologists had predicted.

Admittedly, using psychology to lengthen survival is controversial and has legions of skeptics in medicine, but I wouldn't advise turning your back on any intervention that holds promise for enhancing your life—whether it be emotionally, spiritually, or physically. Your emotional well-being is connected to the entire physiology of your body and may represent one of the newest frontiers in healing.

Discovering more about how your attitudes and beliefs affect your health is the point of this chapter. As we go through this part of the book together, you may discover that you have a deeper reservoir of hope, courage, and optimism than you realize.

FIND YOUR GUARDIAN ANGEL: THE *PUSHKA* STORY

Having doctors whom you trust ties into the ability of the body to heal. I really believe this, not so much because of scientific information I've read, but because I've personally experienced this in my own life in a rather unusual way. My grandmother, affectionately called Nanny Po, who lived to be ninety-eight years old, had in her home what Jewish families call a *pushka*, a small blue-and-white charity box in which you place coins and rolled-up bills that eventually go to support important causes. Not only is it a repository of money, but the family's prayers are bound to every coin as it is put in. Few Jewish homes are without one; it's a way to instill in the family the importance of charity. Nanny Po was the epitome of that spirit. She was full of goodness, and she always looked for the good in other people.

When I went off to college and was studying for my first chemistry exam, Nanny Po called me and learned that I was worried about the test. She reassured me, "Don't worry. I'm going to put some money right now in the *pushka* to assure that you do well on your test. You have nothing to worry about now."

I was pleasantly surprised to find out that I received the second highest grade on that chemistry exam, and I chalked it up to the *pushka*. From that point forward, prior to every semester in college, I would call Nanny Po, and give her a list of my midterms and final exams; she would put money in the *pushka* prior to whatever exam I had coming up. As you might imagine, this was quite an effort, and the *pushka* soon was overflowing with money.

During my junior year in college at the University of Pennsylvania, Nanny Po became seriously ill with a liver abscess and had to be hospitalized. I was facing another big test, but of course, she was unable to put any money in the *pushka*. This was an engineering exam (I was a biomedical engineer as an undergrad), and I incorrectly graphed the numbers for which every question depended on. I believe I received the lowest grade that day on any exam I had ever taken in my entire life. Devastated, I was sure that this happened because it was the first time in three years that I had taken an exam without the comfort of knowing that Nanny Po was simultaneously putting her money in that little blue box.

Thankfully, Nanny Po started feeling better. When she asked about my exams, I had to tell her the truth. She encouraged me to go talk to my professor—which I did, rather reluctantly. I explained to this very seasoned engineering professor that I had a grandmother who was unable to put money in a blue charity box, and this had resulted in my poor performance on the exam. My professor peered over his glasses, stared at me for a few moments in disbelief, and finally said, "Son, I've been at this institution for a very long time. I've never heard a story quite like that. Your concern and love for your grandmother is obvious, although I don't understand the significance of that blue box. However, your story is so good that I'm going to cancel this test grade, and whatever you get on the final test is what you get in the course." And boy, did I ace that final exam (I think Nanny put ten dollars in the *pushka* that day).

Then the story circulated around campus that my grandmother had a "magic box." Friends phoned me, asking to have Nanny Po put money in the *pushka* for them. The thought of that tiny woman giving money to charity for you to succeed was like having a guardian angel by your side. You felt that there was a good, positive, powerful force behind you. Because you believed in it, you somehow believed in yourself and dreams came true! I know mine did, and so did those of many others who believed in the power of hope and goodness.

Why do I tell this story? Because it shows how powerful love, hope, and goodness translate to your belief in yourself, your physician, and your future. If you trust those who are responsible for your medical care and embrace the love of your friends and family, then you, too, can have a guardian angel like Nanny Po by your side and accomplish anything—including solace, hope, and an enhanced sense of well-being.

SEEK AND EMBRACE SUPPORT

Finding sources of emotional support enables you to express your feelings and feel cared for. There is much research showing that belonging to a support group may buffer you against the ravages of stress, improve your quality of life, and enhance your survival

I always recommend joining a cancer support group, where patients can meet and talk about their problems and concerns with other people who have been there. These groups can give you a chance to express your feelings, help you deal with practical issues you're facing such as problems at work or with your family, and help you handle any side effects of treatment. Sometimes, you can't get the support you need from your spouse or your family, and a support group becomes all the more important.

There are different types of support groups. Some are for specific types of cancer only; others are open to people with any type of cancer. Some groups may be for women or men, or specific ethnic groups. Usually, groups are led by other cancer survivors. Other support groups convene online and can be a big help when transportation is a problem. One study found that colon cancer patients enjoyed the anonymity of online participation and felt comfortable "talking" about their treatments. Be wary of Internet groups that offer medical information, however. Online information is not always correct or credible, so never make any changes based on Web advice until you've talked to your doctor.

For some people, support groups don't pan out because hearing sad stories can be depressing. Maybe at this point in your life, you do not want to hear other people's stories about their cancer. That's fine, and very understandable. It is important to be a member of a group that makes you feel better.

If you decide to join a support group, ask your doctor, nurse, social worker, place of worship, or local chapter of the American Cancer Society to help you locate a group near you. There is a list of organizations that can help provide a support group in "Resources" in the back of this book and at the Jay Monahan Center Web site (www.monahancenter.org).

Prior to joining a group, you need to find out who leads the group, how often it meets, how long the meetings last, and the main purpose of the group—to share feelings or solve problems.

After visiting a support group for a few sessions, make sure it meets your needs. Ask yourself:

- *Do I enjoy being a part of the group?*
- *Do I feel uplifted afterward?*
- *Do I get practical advice and hints on how to deal with various cancer issues?*
- *Do I feel as if my views and feelings are respected?*

A yes response to most of those questions means that you'll probably be happy with the support group you've chosen, and that it meets your emotional needs.

GET ASSISTANCE FOR DEPRESSION

Everything about cancer, from its diagnosis to its treatment to dealing with life afterward, can bring on depression. In and out of blue moods, you may feel like you're going crazy. But trust me, you are not going crazy; you are simply going through a crazy time in your life.

If left unchecked, however, depression can progress to a clinical illness that can interfere with healing. When clinically depressed, you may isolate yourself from friends and family—at a time when surrounding yourself with the support of loved ones can actually improve your well-being. Depression can ruin your appetite, too, and you may not get enough calories and nutrients to maintain your weight, fortify your immune system, or enhance healing responses. Depression can also prevent you from getting the restful sleep you need. You may feel anxious, suicidal, and plagued by frequent thoughts of death. In this situation, you need professional help because you are at risk of hurting yourself.

If you think you may be depressed, it's a good idea to ask your physician about medications for depression, anxiety, and sleep problems. There's absolutely nothing wrong with talking to your doctor about this. Taking medications indicates neither a character defect nor a moral flaw. But allowing depression to persist can get in the way of your daily life and your ability to cope emotionally. Antidepressants are very effective for treating clinical depression; they can help you see things in a more rational, positive light and cope more productively with life's stresses.

If anxiety or fear interferes with your ability to enjoy life during or after treatment, then talk to your doctor about a short-acting anti-anxiety medication to help get you through your trying times. *Short-acting* means that the medication does not build up in your body and cause sluggishness or a hungover feeling. Some of the most effective are Xanax and Ativan. They can be taken alone, or are often used in conjunction with antidepressants. For more chronic anxiety, longer-acting agents such as Klonopin may be prescribed.

Both antidepressants and anti-anxiety medications can improve your sleep, but your doctor may also prescribe a sleeping medication to help you get a more restful night's sleep. Currently, there are non-addicting sleeping pills such as Ambien and Sonata available. Ask your doctor about these.

In addition, consider getting professional counseling from a mental health professional (including psychologists and psychiatrists) to help you deal with feelings such as anger, fear, and sadness. Spiritual counseling from your clergy can also help you deal with fear of death or concern for your future or your family's future.

Stress management programs are helpful, too, because they equip you with tools for relaxation and with strategies for gaining control over stress. These programs can teach you how to modify your reactions to stress, so that it is not such a detrimental force in your life.

BE GOOD TO THOSE WHO HELPED YOU

Unfortunately, this often goes unsaid and unrecognized. Tell those who helped you get through this ordeal just how much they mean to you. If you feel that a nurse, technician, or hospital staff member made the extra effort to make you feel comfortable, write a letter to the chief executive officer of the hospital telling him or her who made a difference. Trust me when I say that whoever is named in that letter will know you wrote it.

One thing about having cancer is that your true friends and caring family members surface. Let's face it, it's easy to be a friend when things are good and everybody is having fun. But, when the chips are down, you will find which of your friends and family members are *really* there for you. These are the people you should reach out to and specifically tell how much you appreciate their help. Make a lis of all the family members and friends that were there for you during the worst of times when you needed a hand to hold or were afraid to be alone. For most people, this list is not very long, but it is a very special list indeed. Try to make time to write a note to each of these wonderful people and tell them how much they mean to you. By telling others how they helped you, you are in a way giving back to them. It will feel as good for you to write as it does for those who care about you to read.

FIND MEANING IN YOUR LIFE

Having cancer often causes people to look at their lives in new ways—the "wake-up call" I described earlier. They may change their life goals, rediscover their faith as a source of strength in their lives, or prioritize what they most value in life.

For example, you might change your schedule to spend more time with your family and loved ones. You might begin to realize the importance of the little things in life such as a touch or a smile. You might try to help others by volunteering time or donating to charity. You might put less focus on things like money or your job. You might treat yourself to that car, camera, shoes, or outfit you have always wanted. You might take that expensive vacation or travel to spend time with family and friends and really enjoy their company. In other words, ask yourself:

- *What have I not done that I have always wanted to do?*
- *What have I always wanted to buy?*

- *Who would I like to spend more time with?*
- *Who would I like to speak to more frequently?*
- *Who can I reach out to who might need my help?*
- *Where can I spend some time volunteering?*
- *Which charity can I contribute to?*

Ask yourself these questions, answer them—then do it. This is how you find new meaning in your life and make sense of your cancer experience.

We are all looking for meaning in our lives and by helping others we improve ourselves. As a physician, I have always felt it is a great privilege to be able to help others. You can, too. You might want to help others who are struggling with cancer, since helping others is a path to finding meaning in your life. Many of my patients are asked to appear on TV, talk to the media, or speak with someone recently diagnosed with cancer. You will see that giving something back makes you feel better about yourself. Colorectal cancer patient advocacy groups can always use your help. They are listed in "Resources" in the back of this book. Give them a call.

THE DIFFERENCE BETWEEN PROLONGING LIFE AND PROLONGING DEATH

If someone is terminally ill, finding meaning in life may mean spending his or her final days in relative comfort, as free as possible from the physical and emotional stress often brought on by cancer treatment.

Let me tell you a story about a very brave woman whom I had the pleasure of caring for during her last days of life. When I was chief medical resident, a patient I will refer to as Elizabeth was admitted to New York Hospital with recurrent cancer. Her disease had continued to grow and spread, despite the most aggressive of treatments. When Elizabeth was informed of the situation, she calmly stated that she was ready to be discharged to be with her friends and family. There was no stress in her voice; she knew exactly what she wanted. After Elizabeth left the hospital, we were all silent in unspoken understanding that she did not have long to live. Yet, Elizabeth left us with a smile and died a few days later at home, surrounded by the love of her friends and family. She was truly an exemplary woman in life and in death.

What Elizabeth demonstrated, and what is true in most areas of cancer treatment, is that the quality of a patient's life is far more important than the length of survival. This truth has been slow to sink in with physicians, although understandably so. As doctors, we are taught to treat disease and keep people alive. But sometimes what physicians are doing is not improving or prolonging life, but prolonging death. There is a great deal of suffering attached to that, not only among patients but also among family members who must often stand by, watching a living death.

Fortunately, patients nearing death have a right to choose palliative care to relieve their pain and other symptoms, and I believe this is the best way to achieve quality end-of-life care (see page 166). When the treatment goal changes from prolonging survival to comfort care, patients can end their days with courage, peace, dignity, and comfort.

STAY HOPEFUL

Very central to the healing journey of a person with cancer is the importance of hope. Hope is an inner dynamic force that gives life meaning and helps people live their lives with purpose and dignity, even to the moment of death. Sometimes told in the Jewish faith is the story of the wife whose husband was diagnosed as terminally ill. She consulted her rabbi, who advised her: "First, get the best doctor possible. Second, pray. And third, if the first two fail, do not give up. Hope for a miracle."

As I have stated, miracles can and do happen. Sometimes, however, the hope of a miracle can be dashed when physicians overfocus on a prognosis. Yes, it is true that with cancer, doctors must be up front about the prognosis and give their patients an accurate clinical picture, no matter how discouraging it may be. But we're only working from a table of probabilities. We should never snuff out the last ray of hope a patient may have. Doctors are not gods, and they should never play God by predicting the future. Believe in miracles, and never give up hope.

Understand, too, that hope changes from time to time. It takes on many different forms and is unique to each person. For some, it is the hope for a cure. For others, it is that hope of surviving long enough to attend a daughter's wedding or see a grandchild born. For still others, it is the hope that, despite having cancer, they can live with great joy, meaning, and purpose. For even others, it is the hope of a peaceful death when the time comes.

Sometimes we have to give up hope for one thing, like the hope for a successful treatment, and then we hope for something else, such as reconciling with family members. And so we have different hopes at different stages of treatment and recovery. No matter what is going on in your life, you have the right to hope for whatever is meaningful to you.

My hope for you right now is that you have a deeper, fuller understanding of this disease we call colorectal cancer. I hope it has been eye-opening for you to read and absorb the information I have presented, learning about risk factors, screening, the many ways to prevent this disease, and how to select the right treatment should you ever have to deal with it.

Most of all, I hope you are encouraged and comforted by the knowledge that colorectal cancer is preventable—and it is becoming more curable with each passing year. Someday, I expect to see colorectal cancer drop from the number two spot on the list of cancer killers to the bottom of the list—or fall off the list completely. Colorectal cancer will be tomorrow's memory, and that will be a great day indeed.

While medical science does its part to make that happen, you have yours to do. You know what you must do. Now it's up to you to do it.

Afterword: Into the Future

If you or someone close to you has ever had cancer, or if you have lost a loved one to it, then you know its despair only too well. So I'm sure that you do not wish to see any more lives lost or hurt by this killer disease. Nor do I.

With the huge strides being made in colorectal cancer research just in the last several years, our wish may become more than a dream. Currently, there are more than 400 anticancer drugs in development, many of them designed to fight colorectal cancer—a number up substantially from the roughly 120 test drugs ten years ago. The new gene-based stool tests I mentioned earlier demonstrate just how far we have come in using DNA-specific mutations to detect cancer and polyps. It is hard to believe that DNA was discovered only fifty years ago! And virtual colonoscopies in the future may allow for a less invasive screening test, if the prep can ever be performed "digitally." Meanwhile other medical researchers, including myself, are looking into agents that block the activity of cancer-triggering enzymes—agents that are the closest thing medicine has to prevention in a pill.

Everyone working to fight colorectal cancer knows that there is far more to be done, but the efforts now on the horizon are very promising and encouraging. I don't think there has ever been a more exciting time of discovery in the world of cancer than now.

I know you are thinking: *If so much progress has been made against cancer, then why can't we cure it?*

This is the most common question that I get asked by patients and by anyone who knows I am a doctor interested in cancer. The answer is this: We can, sometimes. If we can't cure the cancer, at least we can treat it as a chronic disease in the same way we treat other chronic, noncancerous illnesses such as diabetes. I have many patients who have survived multiple cancers. In fact, I have one patient who has had six different malignant cancers; she lives a full life.

Unfortunately, advanced cancer is rarely cured. Yet this is the state in which doctors all too often find patients when first diagnosed with cancer. I know this well. My mother was diagnosed with advanced ovarian cancer three years ago. After six cycles of chemotherapy, she was in a complete remission, and it lasted for a year. Not a single cancer cell could be found. But somewhere in her body, a cancer cell was lurking. Her cancer recurred, this time more resistant to chemotherapy. My mother had been just a few cancer cells away from a complete cure.

Imagine how frustrating it has been for me, as the author of this cancer book, to watch my mother's cancer continue to grow, knowing that ovarian cancer can be "cured" if detected early.

Early is the magic word. For ovarian cancer, however, there are no reliable screening techniques, even for early detection. For colorectal cancer, there are.

We know how to beat colorectal cancer through screening—period. But to get everybody to comply with screening means that we have to change the entire way we think about this disease. We practically have to adopt an infectious disease mind-set. What exactly do I mean by that? To cure or eradicate infectious diseases, we vaccinate against the illness. So how do we "vaccinate" against colorectal cancer? Answer: Remove the polyps via a colonoscopy. That is about as close to a vaccination as I know. We would never dream of not vaccinating a child against polio—so why do we not "vaccinate" ourselves from the number two cause of cancer death?

Knowing that we can prevent a cancer, however, isn't much of a comfort to people who are dealing with it, and dying from it. While I sat at her bedside in the hospital producing these words on my laptop, my mother asked me, "Honey, why can't we get rid of my cancer?"

Telling her that we can cure *some* ovarian cancer is neither helpful nor reassuring. You see, from the patient's perspective, despite every scientific discovery, he or she still has cancer. In this situation, we can provide hope, a hand to hold, and comfort, even in the end stages of the disease. As for my mother, I hope that one of the new agents out there may be able to help her. If not, I know that she can be treated to maintain her comfort. But I always hope that she will get better.

If you have cancer, every day is a day of hope. Protect your family by telling them about your illness and encouraging them to discuss prevention with their doctors. If you are fortunate enough to be blessed with good health, treat it as a treasured but fragile possession. Care for it, enjoy it, and certainly do not take it for granted. But, most importantly, don't wait for illness to strike to ask, *Why me?* but prevent it by asking, *Why not me?* Remember: The best person to ensure your good health is not your doctor, but you. That is one piece of lifesaving advice that your doctor may not have told you.

Resources:
Where to Get More Information

GENERAL CANCER RESOURCES

Jay Monahan Center for Gastrointestinal Health
 1315 York Avenue
 New York, New York 10021
 212-746-WELL (746-9355)
 www.monahancenter.org
 A multidisciplinary prevention and treatment center for all gastrointestinal cancers, including colorectal cancer, established at NewYork-Presbyterian Hospital/Weill Cornell Medical Center, in part, through a generous donation from the Entertainment Industry Foundation's National Colorectal Cancer Research Alliance (NCCRA). Named in honor of Jay Monahan, Katie Couric's late husband, the center offers screening and prevention to those who are at risk for colorectal or other GI cancer, and excellence and compassion in care for those who have GI cancer and their families. The Monahan Center's education and outreach program serves to provide information and support for patients and their families, health professionals, and the public on how to reduce your risk for cancer, and how to cope with a diagnosis and treatment.

American Association for Cancer Research
 Public Ledger Building, Suite 816
 150 South Independence Mall West

Philadelphia, Pennsylvania 19106
1-800-477-7127; 215-440-9300
www.aacr.org
Organization of researchers fostering cancer research and providing education to health professionals and the public.

American Cancer Society (ACS)
1599 Clifton Road, NE
Atlanta, Georgia 30329
1-800-ACS-2345 (227-2345)
www.cancer.org
Nonprofit organization funding cancer research and providing a variety of prevention and early-detection programs, as well as cancer information and support to patients, their families, and the general public. Call center is available twenty-four hours a day, seven days a week. Calls are accepted in English or Spanish.

American Institute for Cancer Research
1759 R Street, NW
Washington, D.C. 20009
1-800-843-8114
www.aicr.org
Organization fostering research and education on diet and cancer prevention.

Association of Cancer Online Resources (ACOR)
173 Duane Street, Suite 3A
New York, New York 10013
212-226-5525
www.acor.org
Unique collection of online cancer-related communities designed to provide timely and accurate information in a supportive environment. Provides online mailing lists and Web-based resources.

Cancer Care, Inc.
275 Seventh Avenue
New York, New York 10036

1-800-813-HOPE; 212-302-2400
www.cancercare.org
Provides free counseling, support groups, education and information, and referrals for people with cancer and their families to help them cope with the psychological, social, and financial consequences of cancer. Offers in-person, online, and telephone support groups.

Cancer Hope Network
2 North Road, Suite A
Chester, New Jersey 07930
1-877-HOPENET; 908-879-4039 (inside New Jersey)
www.cancerhopenetwork.org
Offers one-on-one support for people with cancer and their families from trained volunteers who are cancer survivors.

CancerNet
www.cancer.gov
Operated by the National Cancer Institute, this site provides information about cancer, supportive care, screening and prevention, clinical trials, links to other cancer Web sites, and more.

Cancer Research and Prevention Foundation (CRPF)
1600 Duke Street, Suite 500
Alexandria, VA 22314
800-227-2732
703-836-4412
www.preventcancer.org
Advocates the prevention and early detection of cancer through scientific research and education. This organization promotes national colorectal cancer awareness month every March and runs many cancer education programs. Recently, the CRPF toured the "Colossal Colon," a forty foot crawl-through model colon with lifelike polyps and cancer.

**Centers for Disease Control and Prevention (CDC) Division of
Cancer Prevention and Control**
4770 Buford Highway, NE
MS K64
Atlanta, Georgia 30341
1-888-842-6355
www.cdc.gov/cancer
cancerinfo@cdc.gov
Government organization serving to conduct, support, and promote efforts to prevent cancer and to increase early detection of cancer. Develops health communication campaigns, provides cancer
prevention educational materials, and recommends priorities for
health promotion, health education, and cancer risk reduction for
both health professionals and the public.

International Cancer Alliance
4853 Cordell Avenue, Suite 206
Bethesda, Maryland 20814
1-800-422-7361
www.icare.org
Provides user-friendly information on cancer for patients and
their physicians on an ongoing, person-to-person basis.

International Union Against Cancer
3 Rue du Conseil General
1205 Geneva
Switzerland
41-22-809-18-11
www.uicc.org
info@uicc.org
A global cancer organization with members and activities cover-
ing all aspects of cancer control. Provides education and promotes
access to cancer prevention and treatment services throughout the
world.

National Cancer Institute (NCI)
Cancer Information Service (CIS)

9000 Rockville Pike
Bethesda, Maryland 20848
1-800-4-CANCER (422-6237)
www.cancer.gov
The NCI offers a number of cancer programs and services, including the CIS. CIS offers trained cancer staff members who can explain medical terms and issues and provide written materials on many different cancer topics. A CIA specialist can be reached at the toll-free number above or at www.cancer.gov/cis (click on "Live Help").

National Coalition for Cancer Survivorship (NCCS)

1010 Wayne Avenue, Suite 770
Silver Spring, Maryland 20910
1-877-NCCS-YES (622-7937)
www.canceradvocacy.org
info@cansearch.org
Survivor-led cancer advocacy organization, providing information and resources on cancer support, advocacy, and quality-of-life issues, treatment.

COLORECTAL CANCER RESOURCES

National Colorectal Cancer Research Alliance (NCCRA)

www.nccra.org
A nonprofit organization of the Entertainment Industry Foundation (www.eifoundation.org), cofounded by Katie Couric. Serves to raise funds for colorectal cancer research and awareness regarding colorectal cancer screening, prevention, and treatment options.

Colon Cancer Alliance

175 Ninth Avenue
New York, New York 10011
212-627-7451
www.ccalliance.org
Organization of colorectal cancer survivors, caregivers, people

with a genetic predisposition to the disease, and the health care community. Provides patient support services and information. Supports public education, research, and advocacy related to all aspects of colorectal cancer.

Colorectal Cancer Network

P.O. Box 182
Kensington, Maryland 20895
301-879-1500
www.colorectal-cancer.net
ccnetwork@colorectal-cancer.net
Organization of colorectal cancer survivors and their loved ones providing a support network, awareness and screening programs, and legislative actions.

Hereditary Colon Cancer Association

3601 North Fourth Avenue, Suite 201
Sioux Falls, SD 57104
1-800-264-6783
www.hereditarycc.org
Promotes awareness, education, and prevention of hereditary colon cancer and advocates for the need for more research to find better treatments for those who are at risk for or who currently have a hereditary colon cancer. Funds research grants and provides education for health providers, patients, and caregivers.

HEALTH CARE SPECIALTY RESOURCES

American Board of Internal Medicine

510 Walnut Street, Suite 1700
Philadelphia, Pennsylvania 19106
1-800-441-ABIM (2246); 215-446-3500
www.abim.org
Provides an online search for physicians who are board-certified in internal medicine.

American Board of Medical Specialties (ABMS)

1007 Church Street, Suite 404
Evanston, Illinois 60201
847-491-9091
www.abms.org
Provides verification of a physician's board certification by calling
1-866-ASK-ABMS (275- 2267).

American College of Gastroenterology (ACG)

4900B South 31st Street
Arlington, Virginia 22206
703-820-7400
www.acg.gi.org
Organization serving to provide education on gastrointestinal illness and health to health professionals and the public, advocate in the public health and legislative arenas, and promote high standards in medical practice.

American College of Physicians

190 North Independence Mall West
Philadelphia, Pennsylvania 19106
1-800-523-1546
www.acponline.org
Organization dedicated to exchanging the quality and effectiveness of health care by fostering excellence and professionalism in the practice of medicine. Offers a "Home Guide for Advanced Care" on how to manage cancer symptoms and locate help. This guide can be obtained at www.acponline.org/public/homecare.

American College of Surgeons (ACOS)

633 Saint Clair Street
Chicago, Illinois 60611
312-202-5000
www.facs.org
A physician organization dedicated to improving the care of the surgical patient and to safeguarding standards of care in an optimal and ethical practice environment.

American Gastroenterological Association

7910 Woodmont Avenue, Seventh Floor
Bethesda, Maryland 20814
301-654-2055
www.gastro.org
Society of physicians, surgeons, and scientists dedicated to the functions and disorders of the digestive system. Serves to advocate for physician members and their patients, support medical practices and needs, and promote new knowledge in prevention, treatment, and cure of digestive diseases.

American Medical Association (AMA)

515 North State Street
Chicago, Illinois 60610
312-464-5000
www.ama-assn.org
Organization of physicians providing medical news and information for professionals and the public. Provides doctor and medical group locator services.

American Society of Clinical Oncology (ASCO)

1900 Duke Street, Suite 200
Alexandria, Virginia 22314
703-299-0150
www.asco.org; www.plsc.org
asco@asco.org
A national organization of oncologists and researchers that provides cancer information to professionals and the public. Also provides an online list of cancer doctors who are members of ASCO.

American Society of Colon and Rectal Surgeons

85 West Algonquin Road, Suite 550
Arlington Heights, Illinois 60005
847-290-9184
www.fascrs.org
Professional society of surgeons dedicated to promoting science and the treatment of disorders of the colon and rectum. Provides in-

formation for patients on digestive conditions, and colon and rectal surgery. Features a physician locator to identify a board-certified surgeon in your area.

American Society for Gastrointestinal Endoscopy (ASGE)
13 Elm Street
Manchester, Massachusetts 01944
978-526-8330
www.asge.org
Organization of gastroenterologists and surgeons whose members receive specialized training in endoscopic procedures such as colonoscopy. Provides information for patients about diagnosing and treating digestive diseases using endoscopic techniques, and includes physician locator to identify endoscopists in your area.

Association of Community Cancer Centers
11600 Nebel Street, Suite 201
Rockville, MD 20852
www.accc-cancer.org
Organization designed to help oncology professionals provide quality cancer care. Includes a number of excellent resources, including information on cancer drugs, cancer drug reimbursement hotlines, and how to locate a treatment center.

Association of Oncology Social Work (AOSW)
1211 Locust Street
Philadelphia, PA 19107
215-599-6093
www.aosw.org
Organization of professional cancer social workers, dedicated to providing mental and emotional health services to people with cancer, their families, and caregivers. Provides information on AOSW position statements, links to useful resources including a link to the "Cancer Survival Toolbox," free of charge.

National Comprehensive Cancer Network (NCCN)
500 Old York Road, Suite 250

Jenkintown, PA 19046

www.nccn.org

Professional organization, providing clinical guidelines for cancer professionals and for patients and their families. Treatment guidelines for patients are available regarding colorectal cancer and cancer pain, nausea, vomiting, and fatigue.

Oncology Nursing Society

125 Enterprise Drive

Pittsburgh, PA 15275

www.ons.org

Professional organization of registered nurses and other health care providers dedicated to excellence in patient care, education, research, and administration in oncology nursing. Provides information on ONS research, position statements, and resource areas, such as those on cancer-related fatigue and chemotherapy-related nausea and vomiting.

HEALTHCARE QUALITY

Agency for HealthCare Research and Quality (AHRQ)

2101 East Jefferson Street, Suite 501

Rockville, Maryland 20852

301-594-1364

www.ahcpr.gov

Offers a wealth of information on selecting a health plan, doctor, hospital, or a long-term care provider.

Joint Commission on Accreditation of HealthCare Organizations (JCAHO)

1 Renaissance Boulevard

Oakbrook Terrace, Illinois 60181

630-792-5800

www.jcaho.org

Offers an online "Quality Check" service to determine whether a specific facility has been accredited by JCAHO and to view the organization's performance reports.

SPECIAL SUPPORT SERVICES

Corporate Angel Network
1 Loop Road
Westchester County Airport
White Plains, New York 10604
914-328-1313
www.corpangelnetwork.org
Provides free plane transportation for people with cancer going to and from recognized cancer treatment centers by using empty seats aboard corporate aircraft operating on business flights.

Crohn's and Colitis Foundation of America, Inc.
386 Park Avenue South, 17th floor
New York, New York 10016
1-800-932-2423; 212-685-3440
www.ccfa.org
Sponsors research, and provides educational programs and support services for patients with Crohn's disease and colitis, as well as their families.

Kids Konnected
27071 Cabot Road, Suite 102
Laguna Hills, California 92653
1-800-899-2866; 949-582-5443
www.kidskonnected.org
Provides understanding and support to children who have a parent with cancer.

National Patient Air Transport Helpline
P.O. Box 1940
Manassas, Virginia 20108
1-800-296-1217

Makes referrals to charitable, charity-assisted, and special dis-counted patient medical air transport services based on an evalua-tion of patients' needs.

United Ostomy Association
19772 MacArthur Boulevard, Suite 200
Irvine, California 92612
1-800-826-0826; 714-660-8624
www.uoa.org
Provides education, information, support, and advocacy for those who have or will have a colostomy.

CLINICAL TRIALS

National Cancer Institute, National Institute of Health
www.nci.nih.gov/clinicaltrials
Maintains a description of the clinical trial process and a listing of cancer clinical trials.

National Institutes of Health (NIH)
www.clinicaltrials.gov
Provides a listing of current clinical trials searchable by disease.

DRUG INFORMATION

Association of Community Cancer Centers
11600 Nebel Street, Suite 201
Rockville, MD 20852
www.accc-cancer.org
Organization designed to help oncology professionals provide quality cancer care. Includes a number of excellent resources, in-cluding information on cancer drugs, cancer drug reimbursement hotlines, and how to locate a treatment center.

Pharmaceutical Research and Manufacturers of America (PhRMA)

1100 Fifteenth Street, NW

Washington, D.C. 20005

www.phrma.org

Organization of research-based pharmaceutical and biotechnology companies, devoted to inventing medicines that allow patients to live longer, healthier, and more productive lives. Provides information on member drugs, new drugs in development, and a service that helps people identify prescription drug financial assistance programs.

NUTRITION

American Dietetic Association

120 South Riverside Plaza, Suite 2000

Chicago, IL 60606

1-800-877-1600

www.eatright.org

Organization of food and nutrition professionals, providing education and resources. Includes publications by the ADA's Oncology Nutrition Dietetic Practice Group.

Food and Nutrition Information Center

National Agricultural Library

USDA, Room 304

10301 Baltimore Avenue

Beltsville, MD 20705

www.nal.usda.gov/fnic

Part of the U.S. Department of Agriculture. Provides access to information on dietary supplements, food safety, and a section for cancer prevention and survivorship.

U.S. Department of Agriculture (USDA)

14th Street and Independence Avenue, SW

Washington, D.C. 20250

1-888-878-3256

www.nutrition.gov

Government organization providing dietary guidelines, information, and resources.

GENETIC COUNSELING

National Cancer Institute's Cancer Genetics Services Directory

www.cancer.gov/search/genetics_services

1-800-4-CANCER

Provides information on cancer genetics and can help you locate a genetic counselor.

National Society of Genetic Counselors (NSGC)

233 Canterbury Drive

Wallingford, PA 19086

www.nsgc.org

Organization of certified genetic counselors, providing education and referral database to identify certified genetic counselors in your area.

COMPLEMENTARY THERAPIES

National Center for Complementary and Alternative Medicine (NCCAM)

P.O. Box 7923

Gaithersburg, Maryland 20898

1-888-644-6226

www.nccam.nih.gov

info@nccam.nih.gov

Supports research, trains researchers, and provides reliable information about the safety and effectiveness of complementary and alternative medicine.

National Family Caregivers Association

www.nfcacares.org

Organization dedicated to supporting family members caring for a loved one who is ill.

Quackwatch
www.quackwatch.com
This "Guide to Health Fraud, Quackery, and Intelligent Decisions" is maintained by Columbia University Medical Center and includes fact sheets and a glossary of alternative medical practices.

The Wellness Community—National Office
35 East Seventh Street
Cincinnati, Ohio 45202
1-888-793-WELL; 513-421-7111
www.thewellnesscommunity.org
Provides support groups, educational programs, stress management, exercise classes, and social activities at no cost for people with cancer and their families.

Well Spouse Foundation
www.wellspouse.org
Organization dedicated to supporting individuals caring for an ill spouse.

FINANCIAL ISSUES

Cancer Care, Inc.
275 Seventh Avenue
New York, New York 10001
1-800-813-HOPE; 212-302-2400
www.cancercare.org
Organization of social workers that provides counseling, support, and education to people with cancer and their families. Offers guidance on Medicare and Medicaid, and financial assistance for some select services.

Pharmaceutical Research and Manufacturers of America (PhRMA)

1100 Fifteenth Street, NW
Washington, D.C. 20005
1-800-762-4636
www.phrma.org

Organization of pharmaceutical and biochemical companies that provides information and patient assistance programs for patients who cannot afford prescription drug costs.

U.S. Social Security Administration

www.ssa.gov

Provides information and publications for people who have been or will be disabled for six months or longer.

HOSPICE AND ADVANCED ILLNESS CONCERNS

Aging with Dignity

www.agingwithdignity.org

A Web site that focuses on the needs of people who are elderly and those who are nearing the end of life. Includes a document called "Five Wishes" that helps people express how they want to be treated if they are seriously ill and can't speak for themselves.

Calvary Hospital

1740 Eastchester Road
Bronx, NY 10461
718-518-2300
www.calvaryhospital.org

Calvary Hospital is the only fully accredited acute care specialty hospital exclusively providing palliative care for adult advanced cancer patients in the United States. Calvary is committed to kindness, nonabandonment, and the importance of "caring." As the sign says over the main entrance, "A place where life continues . . ."

Growth House

www.growthhouse.org

Provides extensive information about end-of-life issues, palliative care, grief, and bereavement.

Last Acts

www.lastacts.org

A call-to-action program designed to improve care at the end of life, with the goal of helping people and organizations pursue the search for better ways to care for the dying.

National Hospice and Palliative Care Organization (NHPCO)

1700 Diagonal Road, Suite 625
Alexandria, Virginia 22314
1-800-646-6460; 703-837-1500
www.nhpco.org

Oldest and largest nonprofit public benefit organization devoted exclusively to hospice care. Promotes and maintains quality care for terminally ill persons and their families.

Partnership for Caring—National Office

1620 Eye Street NW, Suite 202
Washington, D.C. 20006
1-800-989-9455; 202-296-8071
www.partnershipforcaring.org

National nonprofit organization that brings together individuals and organizations in collaboration to improve how people die in our society. Offers information on living wills, advanced directives, and medical power of attorney.

RESEARCH SOURCES

Medline

www.ncbi.nlm.nih.gov/PubMed/

Provides access to the National Library of Medicine, and includes information about health, a glossary, and the ability to search specific areas of interest.

New York Online Access to Health (NOAH)
www.noah-health.org
This Web site is a project of the City University of New York, the Metropolitan New York Library Council, the New York Academy of Medicine, and the New York Public Library. Includes general resources about prevention, treatment, supportive care, and information sources for colorectal cancer and other diseases.

My Treatment Log

My Health Care Team

(Include your family or primary care physician, gastroenterologist, surgeon, medical oncologist, radiation oncologist, nurse, social worker, dietician, clergy, etc.)

Name	Specialty	Telephone Number
_____	_____	_____
_____	_____	_____
_____	_____	_____
_____	_____	_____
_____	_____	_____
_____	_____	_____
_____	_____	_____
_____	_____	_____
_____	_____	_____
_____	_____	_____

My Hospitals, and/or Clinics or Home Health Agencies

Name	Address	Telephone Number
_____	_____	_____
_____	_____	_____
_____	_____	_____
_____	_____	_____

The Medications I'm Taking

Medication   **When to Take It**

_____   _____

_____   _____

_____   _____

_____   _____

_____   _____

The Tests and Treatments I've Had

Test/Treatment   **Date of Test/Treatment**

_____   _____

_____   _____

_____   _____

_____   _____

_____   _____

_____   _____

_____   _____

_____   _____

Upcoming Appointments

Appointment   **Date**   **Time**

_____   _____   _____

_____   _____   _____

_____   _____   _____

_____   _____   _____

_____   _____   _____

_____   _____   _____

_____   _____   _____

_____   _____   _____

Appointment   Date   Time

Appointment	Date	Time
_____	_____	_____
_____	_____	_____
_____	_____	_____
_____	_____	_____
_____	_____	_____
_____	_____	_____
_____	_____	_____
_____	_____	_____

My Health Insurance

Provider	Plan/Policy Number	Telephone Number
_____	_____	_____
_____	_____	_____
_____	_____	_____

Glossary

Abdominoperineal resection (APR). Surgery to remove cancer located in the lower part of the rectum, where it connects to the anus.

Ablation. A nonsurgical procedure that destroys a tumor by heating it with microwaves, radio frequency, or freezing it.

Adenocarcinoma. A cancerous tumor that grows in the cells lining the inner surface of the colon or rectum area. Adenocarcinoma is not specific to colorectal cancer and can occur in other organ systems (breast, lung, prostate, pancreas, etc.).

Adenomatous polyp. A growth of cells that line the inside of the colon or rectum. Adenomatous polyps may develop into cancer if not removed.

Adjuvant therapy. A treatment that is used in addition to the main treatment. It usually involves chemotherapy, radiation, or immunotherapy following surgery in order to cure the disease or stop its progression.

Alternative therapy. A treatment that is considered unconventional compared to standard medical treatments and that is often used in place of standard therapy. (See "complementary therapy.")

Anastomosis. In colorectal operations, the site where two structures are surgically joined together. For example, after removal of a part of the colon that is malignant, the ends of the colon are rejoined at a site called the anastamosis.

Antimetabolite drugs. Chemotherapy agents that disrupt DNA production, which in turn prevents cell division and growth of tumors.

Antioxidants. Nutrients—found mainly in foods—that protect the body against damage from destructive molecules known as free radicals.

Apoptosis. The gene-controlled process of programmed cell death in which cells die at a specific time.

Average risk. Someone with no family history or increased risk of colorectal cancer.

Benign. Not cancerous.

Biopsy. Microscopic examination of tissues or cells removed from the body.

Cancer. An alteration of normal cells that causes uncontrolled growth and spreading of these cells.

Cancer vaccine. A substance made from pieces of tumors or cancer proteins that works by causing the immune system to recognize and attack cancer cells.

Carcinoma in situ. The earliest stage of cancer in which the tumor is confined to the most superficial site where it started.

Chemotherapy. A cancer treatment that uses specific drugs, either intravenously or orally, to destroy cancerous cells.

Clinical trials. Studies that compare a standard treatment with a newly developed treatment. Clinical trials are usually done in three phases. Phase I tests the dose and safety of the treatment on a small number of patients. Phase II studies the effectiveness of the treatment and usually involves a larger sample of people. Phase III provides in-depth information about the effectiveness and safety, by comparing experimental treatment with the standard treatment.

Colectomy. The surgical removal of all or part of the colon.

Colonoscopy. An examination of the colon using a long flexible scope and camera to look for polyps, cancer, and diseases of the colon and rectum.

Colorectal. Pertaining to any area in the colon or the rectum.

Colostomy. An opening (stoma) from the colon onto the skin of the abdomen so that stool can be eliminated. It is created during surgical procedure that routes the colon to this opening and can be temporary or permanent. The opening is covered by a bag to collect the fecal matter.

Combination chemotherapy. The use of two or more drugs to treat cancer.

Complementary therapy. Therapies that are used in addition to standard treatments. The goals of complementary therapies are usually to relieve symptoms of cancer, relieve the side effects of cancer treatment, reduce stress, and enhance a patient's sense of well-being.

Computerized tomography (CT or CAT scan). An imaging procedure that combines X rays with a computer to produce detailed pictures of cross sections of the body and organs.

COX-1, COX-2. Enzymes found in cells that trigger various processes in the body, including inflammation.

COX inhibitors. Agents such as aspirin and other nonsteroid anti-inflammatory drugs that interfere with the activity of COX-1 and COX-2 enzymes. The newer COX-2 inhibitors, celecoxib (Celebrex) and rofecoxib (Vioxx), may play a role in cancer prevention.

Cryosurgery. The use of extreme cold to freeze and destroy cancer cells.

Digital rectal examination. An exam used to detect cancer in which a doctor inserts a gloved lubricated finger into the rectum and probes for abnormalities.

Double contrast barium enema. A screening test that involves the use of X rays and barium (called the contrast medium) to look for polyps, cancer, inflammatory bowel disease, or other abnormalities in the colon and rectum.

Dukes-Kirklin. A system used for staging colorectal cancer that describes the extent of the disease in a patient by letter designation (A, B, C or D).

Endocavitary radiation therapy. A form of radiation therapy for treating cancer in which the radiation beam is aimed through the anus into the rectum.

External beam radiation. A procedure in which radiation is focused from a source outside the body on the area where the cancer is located.

Familial adenomatous polyposis (FAP). A heredity condition that will result in colorectal cancer. People with FAP develop thousands of polyps in their colon or rectum and at least one will turn malignant if preventive surgery is not done.

Fecal occult blood test (FOBT). A screening test for colon or rectal cancer that detects microscopic (occult) blood in the stool. It can be performed at home.

Gastroenterology. A specialty of internal medicine that focuses on treating diseases of the digestive system. This includes the gastrointestinal tract and associated organs such as the liver and pancreas.

Gene. A segment of DNA that holds information on hereditary traits such as hair and eye color and height, as well as susceptibility to certain diseases.

Genetic testing. Special tests performed to see if a person has specific gene alterations. It is recommended only for those with specific types of family cancer history. Genetic counseling is a component of genetic testing.

Hereditary nonpolyposis colorectal cancer (HNPCC). A hereditary condition that is a risk factor for developing polyps, colorectal cancer, and other associated cancers.

High risk. A category of risk meaning that someone's chance of getting a disease is higher than that of the general population.

Hyperplastic polyps. Benign growths in the colon or rectum. These polyps are *not* thought to be potentially precancerous like the adenomatous polyps.

Infusion. Slow and/or prolonged delivery of a drug or fluids.

Intravenous (IV). Into a vein.

Laparoscopy. A less invasive surgical procedure in which the surgeon inserts a long slender camera through a very small incision. It is used to do some types of surgery for colorectal cancer.

Low anterior resection (LAR). Surgery that removes cancer and the healthy tissue around it near the upper part of the rectum, where it connects to the sigmoid colon.

Lymph nodes. A part of the immune system consisting of small bean-shaped organs that filter out germs and abnormal cells.

Magnetic resonance imaging (MRI). A diagnostic imaging method that combines magnetic fields, radio waves, and a computer to produce a detailed cross-sectional picture of the inside of the body.

Malignant. Cancerous.

Margin. The edge of removed tissue. A negative surgical margin means that there was no cancer near the area from which the tissue was removed. A positive surgical margin indicates that cancer cells exist at the outer edge of the tissue removed; this is usually a sign that some cancer may remain in the body.

Medical oncology. A subspecialty of internal medicine that employs chemotherapy, as well as nonradiation and nonsurgical treatments, to treat cancer.

Metastasis. The spread of cancer cells from the primary (original) site to another site or sites in the body.

Neoadjuvant therapy. Treatment that is administered prior to the primary treatment of surgery or radiation. Radiation may also be a part of neoadjuvant therapy for rectal cancer.

Oncogenes. Genes that promote cell growth and multiplication that are normally present in all cells. Oncogenes may become altered, causing cells to grow too rapidly and form tumors.

Palliative therapy. Treatment to relieve the symptoms caused by cancer and help people live more comfortably.

Phytochemicals. Natural chemicals in fruits, vegetables, and grains that act as antioxidants, and exert other beneficial and protective effects in the body.

Polyp. A flat or mushroom-shaped growth on the lining of the colon.

Polypectomy. Removal of a polyp. This is usually performed during a colonoscopy.

Prognosis. A prediction explaining the likely outcome of a disease or chance of survival in a particular patient.

Radiation oncology. A specialty that uses various forms of radiation to treat cancer.

Radiation therapy. A treatment that uses high doses of radiation to treat or control cancer.

Recurrence. Cancer that has returned after treatment. *Local recurrence* means that it has returned to the original site. *Regional re-*

currence means that it has returned to the lymph nodes or to tissues near the original site. *Distant recurrence* is the term used to describe cancer that has metastasized, or spread, to other organs or tissues.

Remission. A period of time when the cancer responds well to treatment or is under control.

Resection. Surgery that removes part of or all of an organ or other structure.

Segmental resection. Surgery that removes the cancer and the length of healthy tissue surrounding the cancer, as well as nearby lymph nodes, then reconnects the remaining sections of the colon.

Sigmoidoscopy. A test utilizing a flexible tube and camera that enables a doctor to view the lower third of the colon and rectum.

Stage. A classification of the extent of cancer.

Surgical oncology. A surgical subspecialty that focuses on treating cancer surgically.

Survival rate. The percentage of survivors with no sign of disease within a certain period of time after diagnosis or treatment. For cancer, a five-year survival rate is often given. This is strictly a statistical number to help guide therapy.

TNM system. A staging system for cancer that gives three key pieces of information: T refers to the size of the tumor, N describes how far the cancer has spread to nearby nodes, and M shows whether the cancer has spread or metastasized to other organs of the body. Letters or numbers following the T, N, and M designation give more details about each of these factors.

Tumor. An abnormal growth of cells that can be benign or malignant.

Ultrasound. A painless, noninvasive imaging method that uses high-frequency sound waves to locate and measure tumors and other abnormal growths in the body.

References

CHAPTER 1: THE TRUTH ABOUT COLORECTAL CANCER

American Cancer Society. 2003. "How Many People Get Colorectal Cancer?" Online: www.cancer.org.

Editor. 1999. "Harvard Report on Cancer Prevention." *Cancer Causes and Control* 10: 167–180.

Kopp-Hoolihan, L. 2001. "Prophylactic and Therapeutic Uses of Probiotics: A Review." *Journal of the American Dietetic Association* 101: 229–238.

CHAPTER 2: RISK FACTORS: WHO GETS COLORECTAL CANCER AND WHY?

American Cancer Society. 2003. "What Are the Risk Factors for Colon and Rectum Cancer?" Online: www.cancer.org.

Bajanda, L. 2000. "The Effects of Alcohol Consumption Upon the Gastrointestinal Tract." *The American Journal of Gastroenterology* 95: 3374–3382.

Bostick, R.M. 2000. "Nutrition and Colon Cancer Prevention." *Cancer & Nutrition: Prevention and Treatment* 4: 67–86.

Driver, H.E., et al. 1987. "Alcohol and Human Cancer (Review)." *Anticancer Research* 7: 309–320.

Geboes, K. 2000. "Ulcerative Colitis and Malignancy." *Acta-Gastroenterologia Belgica* 63: 279–283.

Giovannucci, E. et al. 1994. Intake of fat, meat, and fiber in relation to risk of colon cancer in men. *Cancer Research* 54: 2390–2397.

———. "Multivitamin Use, Folate, and Colon Cancer in Women in the Nurses' Health Study." *Annals of Internal Medicine* 129: 517–524.

———. 1996. "Physical Activity, Obesity, and Risk of Colorectal Adenoma in Women (United States)." *Cancer Causes and Control* 7: 253–263.

Goldbohm, R.A., et al. 1994. "Prospective Study on Alcohol Consumption and the Risk of Cancer of the Colon and Rectum in the Netherlands." *Cancer Causes and Control* 5: 95–104.

Hall, L.L. 2000. "Preventing Colon Cancer." *FDA Consumer*, November–December, pp. 14–18.

Hill, M.J. 1999. "Mechanisms of Diet and Colon Carcinogenesis." *European Journal of Cancer Prevention* 8 Supplement 1: S95–S98.

Jemel, A., et al. 2003. "Cancer Statistics, 2003." *CA: A Cancer Journal for Clinicians* 53: 5–26.

Knekt, P., et al. 1999. "Risk of Colorectal and Other Gastro-intestinal Cancers After Exposure to Nitrate and N-nitroso Compounds: A Follow-up Study." *International Journal of Cancer* 15: 852–856.

Lynch, H.T., et a;. 2003. "Hereditary Colorectal Cancer." *New England Journal of Medicine* 348: 919–932.

Ma, J., et al. 2000. "A Prospective Study of Plasma Levels of Insulin-like Growth Factor I (IGF-I) and IGF-Binding Protein-3, and Colorectal Cancer Risk Among Men." *Growth Hormone & IGF Research* 10 Supplement A: S28–S29.

Schoen, R.E., et al. 1999. "Increased Blood Glucose and Insulin, Body Size, and Incident Colorectal Cancer." *Journal of National Cancer Institute* 91: 1147–1154.

Slattery, M.L., et al. 2000. "Associations between Cigarette Smoking,

Lifestyle Factors, and Microsatellite Instability in Colon Tumors." *Journal of the National Cancer Institute* 92: 1831–1836.

Slattery, M.L., et al. 2001. "Dietary Intake and Microsatellite Instability in Colon Tumors." *International Journal of Cancer* 93: 601–607.

Traverso, G., et al. 2002. "Detection of APC Mutations in Fecal DNA from Patients with Colorectal Tumors." *New England Journal of Medicine* 346: 311–320.

Trimbath, J.D., et al. "Review Article: Genetic Testing and Counseling for Hereditary Colorectal Cancer." *Alimentary Pharmacology & Therapeutics* 16: 1843–1857.

Vaisman, N., et al. 2002. "The role of Nutrition and Chemoprevention in Colorectal Cancer: From Observations to Expectations." *Best Practice & Research, Clinical Gastroenterology* 16: 201–217.

CHAPTER 3: COLONOSCOPY: YOUR MOST POWERFUL WEAPON AGAINST COLORECTAL CANCER

Editor. 1999. "Harvard Report on Cancer Prevention." *Cancer Causes and Control* 10: 167–180.

Editor. 2001. "Low Residue Foods Replace Liquid Diet for Improved Patient Compliance and Tolerance." *Business Wire,* September 10. News release.

Verghese, V.J., et al. 2002. "Low-Salt Bowel Cleansing Preparation (LoSo Prep) as a Preparation for Colonoscopy: a pilot study." *Alimentary Pharmacology & Therapeutics* 16: 1327–1331.

CHAPTER 4: OTHER SCREENING TECHNOLOGIES

American Cancer Society and National Comprehensive Cancer Network. 2002. "Colon and Rectal Cancer: Treatment Guidelines for Patients." Version II.

Baltrusch, H.J., et al. 1991. "Stress, Cancer and Immunity: New Developments in Biopsychosocial and Psychoneuroimmunologic Research." *Acta Neurologica* 13: 315–327.

Burgess, C., et al. 1988. "Psychological Response to Cancer Diagnosis— II. Evidence for Coping Styles (Coping Styles and Cancer Diagnosis)." *Journal of Psychosomatic Research* 32: 263–272.

College of American Pathologists Protocol for polypectomy and for Surgical Pathology.

Greer, S., et al. 1979. "Psychological Response to Breast Cancer: Effect on Outcome." *Lancet* 2: 785–787.

Hoodin, F. 2003. "A Systematic Review of Psychosocial Factors Affecting Survival After Bone Marrow Transplantation." *Psychosomatics* 44: 181–195.

Pickhardt, P.J., et. al. 2003 "Computed Tomographic Virtual Colonosocopy to screen for Colorectal Neoplasia in Asymptomatic Adults." *The New England Journal of Medicine.* 349: 2191–2200.

Ponz de Leon, M. 2002. *Colorectal Cancer.* New York: Springer.

CHAPTER 5: EAT SMART, LIVE RIGHT

Bandaru, S., et al. 2000. "Preventive Potential of Wheat Bran Fractions Against Experimental Colon Carcinogenesis: Implications for Human Colon Cancer Prevention." *Cancer Research* 60: 4792–4797.

Birchard, K. 2001. "Fibre Does Cut Bowel Cancer Risk: Study." *Medical Post,* August 21. Online: www.elibrary.com.

Bonithon-Kopp, C., et al. 2000. "Calcium and Fibre Supplementation in Prevention of Colorectal Adenoma Recurrence: A Randomized Intervention Trial." *The Lancet* 356: 1300–1306.

Bostick, R.M. 2000. "Nutrition and Colon Cancer Prevention." *Cancer & Nutrition: Prevention and Treatment* 4: 67–86.

Bowes and Church's Food Values of Portions Commonly Used. 1998. 17th ed., revised by J. Pennington. Philadelphia: Lippincott Williams and Wilkins.

Brustman, B. 2000. "Healthy Lifestyles, Regular Screenings Would Cut U.S. Colon Cancer Morbidity in Half." January 20. Online: www.re-searchmatters.harvard.edu.

Butler, L., et al. 2003. "Heterocyclic Amines, Meat Intake, and Association with Colon Cancer in a Population-Based Study." *American Journal of Epidemiology* 157: 434–445.

Editor. 2002. *Taking a Closer Look at Phytochemicals.* Washington, D.C. The American Institute for Cancer Research.

Fernandez, E., et al. 1999. "Fish Consumption and Cancer Risk." *American Journal of Clinical Nutrition* 170: 85–90.

Fuchs, C.S., et al. 1999. "Dietary Fiber and the Risk of Colon Cancer and Adenoma in Women." *The New England Journal of Medicine* 340: 169–176.

Giovannucci, E. 1995. "Insulin and Colon Cancer." *Cancer Causes and Control* 6: 164–179.

———.1994. "Intake of Fat, Meat, and Fiber in Relation to Risk of Colon Cancer in Men." *Cancer Research* 54: 2390–2397.

———. 1996. "Physical Activity, Obesity, and Risk of Colorectal Adenoma in Women (United States)." *Cancer Causes and Control* 7: 253–263.

———. Relationship of Diet to Risk of Colorectal Adenoma in Men." *Journal of the National Cancer Institute* 84: 91–98.

Harvard Center for Cancer Prevention. 2003. "Colon Cancer Risk List." Online: www.yourcancerrisk.harvard.edu.

La Vecchia, C., et al. 1993. "Refined-Sugar Intake and the Risk of Colorectal Cancer in Humans." *International Journal of Cancer* 55: 386–389.

Lewis, C., et al. 1999. "Health Claims and Observational Human Data: Relation between Dietary Fat and Cancer. *American Journal of Clinical Nutrition* 69 Supplement: 1357S–1364S.

Lipkin, M., et al. 1999. "Dietary Factors in Human Colorectal Cancer." *Annual Review of Nutrition* 19: 545–586.

Michels, K.B., et al. 2000. "Prospective Study of Fruit and Vegetable Consumption and Incidence of Colon and Rectal Cancers." *Journal of the National Cancer Institute* 92: 1740–1752.

Orellana, C. 2002. "Bile Acids, Oxidative Stress, and Colon Cancer." *Lancet Oncology* 3: 588.

Owen, R., et al. 2000. "Olive-Oil Consumption and Health: The Possible Role of Antioxidants." *Lancet* 1: 107–112.

Perdignon, G., et al. "Role of Yoghurt in the Prevention of Colon Cancer." *European Journal of Clinical Nutrition* 46: S65–S-68.

Rao, C.V., et al. 1998. "Chemopreventive Effect of Squalene on Colon Cancer." *Carcinogenesis* 19: 287–290.

Schatzin, A., et al. 2000. "Lack of Effect of a Low-Fat, High-Fiber Diet on the Recurrence of Colorectal Adenomas." *New England Journal of Medicine* 342: 1149–1155.

Shannon, J., et al. 1996. "Relationship of Food Groups and Water Intake to Colon Cancer Risk." *Cancer Epidemiology, Biomarkers and Prevention* 5: 495–502.

Slattery, M.L., et al. 2000. "Carotenoids and Colon Cancer." *American Journal of Clinical Nutrition* 71: 575–582.

Slattery, M.L., et al. 2002. "Physical Activity and Colon Cancer: Confounding or Interaction?" *Medicine and Science in Sports and Exercise* 34: 913–919.

Slattery, M.L., et al. "Trans-Fatty Acids and Colon Cancer." *Nutrition and Cancer* 39: 170–175.

Tuck, K.L., et al. 2002. "Major Phenolic Compounds in Olive Oil: Metabolism and Health Effects." *Journal of Nutritional Biochemistry* 13: 636–644.

VanDuyn, M., et al. 2000. "Overview of the Health Benefits of Fruit and Vegetable Consumption for the Dietetics Professional." *Journal of the American Dietetic Association* 100: 1511–1521.

Weisburger, J.H., et al. 1983. "Bile Acids, But Not Neutral Sterols, Are

Tumor Promoters in the Colon in Man and in Rodents." *Environmental Health Perspective* 50: 101–107.

Weisburger, J.H. 1997. "Dietary Fat and Risk of Chronic Disease: Mechanistic Insights from Experimental Studies." *Journal of the American Dietetic Association* 97: S16–23.

Willet, W.C. 1999. "Convergence of Philosophy and Science: The Third International Congress on Vegetarian Nutrition." *American Journal of Clinical Nutrition* 70: 434S–438S.

Wollowski, I., et al. 2001. "Protective Role of Probiotics and Prebiotics in Colon Cancer." *American Journal of Clinical Nutrition* 73 Supplement. 451S–455S.

CHAPTER 6: CURB COLORECTAL CANCER: SUPPLEMENTS AND CHEMOPREVENTION

Baron, J.A., et al. 2003. "A Randomized Trial of Aspirin to Prevent Colorectal Adenomas." *New England Journal of Medicine* 348: 891–899.

Bostick, R.M. 2000. "Nutrition and Colon Cancer Prevention." *Cancer & Nutrition: Prevention and Treatment* 4: 67–86.

Chauhan, D.P. 2002. "Chemotherapeutic Potential of Curcumin for Colorectal Cancer." *Current Pharmaceutical Design* 8: 1695–1706.

Choi, S.W., et al. 2002. "Folate Status: Effects on Pathways of Colorectal Carcinogenesis." *Journal of Nutrition* 132: 2413S–2418S.

Editor. 2002. "The Latest on Postmenopausal Hormones." *NHS News,* autumn, p. 1.

Garland, C.F., et al. 1999. "Calcium and Vitamin D: Their Potential Roles in Colon and Breast Cancer Prevention." *Annals of the New York Academy of Science* 889: 107–119.

Gescher, A., et al. 2001. "Cancer Chemoprevention by Dietary Constituents: A Tale of Failure and Promise." *Lancet Oncology* 2: 371–379.

Giovannucci, E. 2002. "Epidemiologic Studies of Folate and Colorectal Neoplasia: A Review." *Journal of Nutrition* 132: 2350S–2355S.

———. "Multivitamin Use, Folate, and Colon Cancer in Women in the Nurses' Health Study." *Annals of Internal Medicine* 129: 517–524.

Holt, P.R., et al. 1998. "Modulation of Abnormal Colonic Epithelial Cell Proliferation and Differentiation by Low-Fat Dairy Foods: A Randomized Controlled Trial." *Journal of the American Medical Association* 280: 1074–1079.

Lieberman, D.A., et al. 2003. "Risk Factors for Advanced Colonic Neoplasia and Hyperplastic Polyps in Asymptomatic Individuals." *Journal of the American Medical Association* 290: 2959–2967.

Lipkin, M., et al. 1985. "Effect of Added Dietary Calcium on Colonics Epithelial-Cell Proliferation in Subjects at High Risk for Familial Colonics Cancer." *New England Journal of Medicine* 28: 1381–1384.

Mouzas, I.A., et al. 1998. "Chemoprevention of Colorectal Cancer in Inflammatory Bowel Disease? A Potential Role for Folate." *Italian Journal of Gastroenterology and Hepatology* 30: 421–425.

Nelson, H., et al. "Postmenopausal Hormone Replacement Therapy: Scientific Review." *Journal of the American Medical Association* 288: 872–881.

Phillips, R.K., et al. 2002. "A Randomised, Double Blind, Placebo Controlled Study of Celecoxib, a Selective Cyclooxygenase 2 Inhibitor, on Duodenal Polyposis in Familial Adenomatous Polyposis." *Gut* 50: 857–860.

Sandler, R.S., et al. 2002. "A Randomized Trial of Aspirin to Prevent Colorectal Adenomas in Patients with Previous Colorectal Cancer." *New England Journal of Medicine* 348: 883–890.

Sansom, C. 2001. "Curry Component May Be Chemopreventive for Colon Cancer." *Lancet Oncology* 2: 67.

Sheehan, K., et al. 1999. "The Relationship between Cyclooxygenase-2 Expression and Colorectal Cancer." *Journal of the American Medical Association* 282: 1254–1257.

Slattery, M.L., et al. 1998. "Vitamin E and Colon Cancer: Is There an Association?" *Nutrition and Cancer* 30: 201–206.

Sturmer, T., et al. 1998. "Aspirin Use and Colorectal Cancer: Post-Trial Follow-up Data from the Physicians' Health Study." *Annals of Internal Medicine* 128: 713–720.

Thun, M., et al. 1991. "Aspirin Use and Reduced Risk of Fatal Colon Cancer." *New England Journal of Medicine* 325: 1593–1596.

Thun, M., et al. 2002. "Nonsteroidal Anti-inflammatory Drugs as Anti-cancer Agents: Mechanistic, Pharmacologic, and Clinical Issues." *Journal of the National Cancer Institute* 94: 252–266.

Vaisman, N., et al. 2002. "The Role of Nutrition and Chemoprevention in Colorectal Cancer: From Observations to Expectations." *Best Practice & Research, Clinical Gastroenterology* 16: 201–217.

Wargovich, M.J. 2001. "Colon Cancer Chemoprevention with Ginseng and Other Botanicals." *Journal of Korean Medical Science* 16: S81–S86.

Whiting, S.J., et al. 1997. "Calcium Supplementation." *Journal of the American Academy of Nurse Practitioners* 9: 187–192.

Wu, K., et al. 2002. "Calcium Intake and Risk of Colon Cancer in Women and Men." *Journal of the National Cancer Institute* 94: 437–446.

CHAPTER 7: GETTING A DIAGNOSIS: UNDERSTANDING PATHOLOGY AND STAGING

College of American Pathologists. 2003. "Colon and Rectum Protocols." Online: www.cap.org.

CHAPTER 8: DEALING WITH YOUR DIAGNOSIS AND CHOOSING DR. RIGHT

American Board of Colon and Rectal Surgery. 2003. "Definition of a Board Certified Colon and Rectal Surgeon." Online: www.abcrs.org.

American Board of Internal Medicine. 2003. "Certification." Online: www.abim.org.

American Board of Medical Specialties. 2003. "What Is the ABMS?" Online: www.abms.org.

American Board of Radiology. 2003. "About the Board." Online: www.theabr.org.

American Board of Surgery. 2003. "Which Medical Specialist for You?" Online: www.abms.org.

American Hospital Association. 2003. "A Patient's Bill of Rights." Online: www.hospitalconnect.com.

Hannan, E.L., et al. 2002. "The Influence of Hospital and Surgeon Volume on In-Hospital Mortality and Colectomy, Gastrectomy, and Lung Lobectomy in Patients with Cancer." *Surgery* 131: 6–15.

Harmon, J.W., et al. 1999. "Hospital Volume Can Serve as a Surrogate for Surgeon Volume for Achieving Excellent Outcomes in Colorectal Resection." *Annals of Surgery* 230: 404–411; discussion 411–413.

National Cancer Institute. 2003. The National Cancer Institute Cancer Centers Program. Online: cis.nci.nih.gov.

Schrag, D., et al. 2000. "Influence of Hospital Procedure Volume on Outcomes Following Surgery for Colon Cancer." *Journal of the American Medical Association* 284: 3028–3035.

Singh, K. K., et al. 1997. "Audit of Colorectal Cancer Surgery by Nonspecialist Surgeons." *British Journal of Surgery* 84: 343–347.

Wallerstein, N. 1992. "Powerlessness, Empowerment, and Health: Implications for Health Promotion Programs." *American Journal of Health Promotion* 6: 197–205.

CHAPTER 9: WHEN SURGERY IS THE ANSWER

American Cancer Society. 2003. "Surgery." Online: www.cancer.org.

American Cancer Society and National Comprehensive Cancer Network. 2002. "Colon and Rectal Cancer: Treatment Guidelines for Patients." Version II.

American Society of Colon and Rectal Surgeons. 2003. "Follow-Up and Evaluation After Surgery for Colon Cancer." Online: www.fascrs.org.

Lacy, A.M., et al. 2002. "Laparoscopy-Assisted Colectomy Versus Open Colectomy for Treatment of Nonmetastatic Colon Cancer: A Randomized Trial." *Lancet* 359: 2224–2229.

Lian-Xin, L., et al. 2003. "Current Treatment for Liver Metastases from Colorectal Cancer." *World Journal of Gastroenterology* 9: 193–200.

Ponz de Leon, M. 2002. *Colorectal Cancer.* New York: Springer.

Richard, M. 2001. "Laparoscopy for Colon Cancer." *Surgical Oncology Clinics of North America* 10: 579–597.

CHAPTER 10: IF YOU NEED CHEMOTHERAPY OR RADIATION THERAPY

American Cancer Society. 2003. "Chemotherapy." Online: www.cancer.org.

American Cancer Society. 2003. "Handling the Side Effects of Treatment." Online: www.cancer.org.

American Cancer Society. 2003. "Understanding Radiation Therapy: A Guide for Patients and Families." Online: www.cancer.org.

American Cancer Society and National Comprehensive Cancer Network. 2002. "Colon and Rectal Cancer: Treatment Guidelines for Patients." Version II.

Chau, I., et al. 2002. "Chemotherapy in Colorectal Cancer: New Options and New Challenges." *British Medical Bulletin* 64: 159–180.

Douillard, J.Y. 2000. "Irinotecan and High-Dose Fluorouracil/Leucovorin for Metastatic Colorectal Cancer." *Oncology* 14 Supplement: 51–55.

Editor. 2002. "Eloxatin (Oxaliplatin for Injection)." *Clinician Reviews,* November. Online: www.findarticles.com.

Hoff, P.M., et al. 2001. "Comparison of Oral Capecitabine Versus Intravenous Fluorouracil Plus Leucovorin as First-Line Treatment in 605 Patients with Metastatic Colorectal Cancer: Results of a Randomized Phase III Study. *Journal of Clinical Oncology* 19: 2282–2292.

Lian-Xin, L., et al. 2003. "Current Treatment for Liver Metastases from Colorectal Cancer." *World Journal of Gastroenterology* 9: 193–200.

Ponz de Leon, M. 2002. *Colorectal Cancer.* New York: Springer.

Stubbs, R.S., et al. 2001. "Selective Internal Radiation Therapy (SIRT) with 90Yttrium Microspheres for Extensive Colorectal Cancer Metastases. *Hepatogastroenterology* 48: 333–337.

CHAPTER 11: COMPLEMENTARY THERAPIES FOR COLORECTAL CANCER

American Cancer Society. 2000. "American Cancer Society's Guide to Complementary and Alternative Methods." Online: www.cancer.org.

Barrows, K., et al. 2002. "Mind-Body Medicine. An Introduction and Review of the Literature." *The Medical Clinics of North America* 86: 11–31.

Burish, T.G., et al. 1992. "Psychological Techniques for Controlling the Adverse Side Effects of Cancer Chemotherapy: Findings from a Decade of Research." *Journal of Pain and Symptom Management* 7: 287–301.

Cassileth, B.R. 1999. "Evaluating Complementary and Alternative Therapies for Cancer Patients." *CA: A Cancer Journal for Clinicians* 49: 362–375.

Editor. 2002. "Yoga May Offer Benefits to Patients with Cancer." *Clinical Journal of Oncology Nursing* 6: 253.

Ernst, E. 2001. "A Primer of Complementary and Alternative Medicine Commonly Used by Cancer Patients." *Medical Journal of Australia* 174: 88–92.

Ferrell-Terry, A.T., et al. 1993. "The Use of Therapeutic Massage as a Nursing Intervention to Modify Anxiety and the Perception of Cancer Pain." *Cancer Nursing* 16: 93–101.

Ironson, G., et al. 1999. "Massage Therapy Is Associated with Enhancement of the Immune System's Cytotoxic Capacity." *International Journal of Neuroscience* 84: 205–217.

Lan, C., et al. 2002. "Tai Chi Chuan: An Ancient Wisdom on Exercise and Health Promotion." *Sports Medicine* 32: 217–224.

Thomas, E.M., et al. 2000. "Nonpharmacological Interventions with Chronic Cancer Pain in Adults." *Cancer Control* 7: 157–164.

CHAPTER 12: LIFE AFTER COLORECTAL CANCER

American Cancer Society. 2003. "Cancer Treatment's Effect on Female Sexual Desire and Response." Online: www.cancer.org.

American Cancer Society. 2003. "Coping with Cancer in Everyday Life." Online: www.cancer.org.

American Cancer Society. 2003. "Ways of Dealing with Sexual Problems." Online: www.cancer.org.

American Cancer Society. 2003. "What Happens After Treatment?" Online: www.cancer.org.

Batty, D. 2000. "Does Physical Activity Prevent Cancer?" *British Medical Journal* 321: 1424–1425.

DeCosse, J.J., et al. 1997. "Quality-of-Life-Management of Patients with Colorectal Cancer." *CA:A Cancer Journal for Clinicians* 47: 198–206.

Graham, S. 1986. "Hypotheses Regarding Caloric Intake in Cancer Development." *Cancer* 58 Supplement 8: 1814–1817.

Jacobs, E.T., et al. 2002. "Intake of Supplemental and Total Fiber and Risk of Colorectal Adenoma Recurrence in the Wheat Bran Trial." *Cancer Epidemiology, Biomarkers & Prevention* 11: 906–914.

Lebeau, D. 1998. "Chemoprevention Controversies Continue." *Lancet* 352: 1683.

Lyon, J.L., et al. 1987. "Energy Intake: Its Relationship to Colon Cancer Risk." *Journal of the National Cancer Institute* 78: 853–861.

Maeda, M., et al. 1998. "Alcohol Consumption Enhances Liver Metastasis in Colorectal Carcinoma Patients." *Cancer* 83: 1483–1488.

Ponz de Leon, M. 2002. *Colorectal Cancer.* New York: Springer.

Schatzkin, A., et al. 2000. "Lack of Effect of a Low-Fat, High-Fiber Diet on the Recurrence of Colorectal Adenomas: Polyp Prevention Trial Study Group." *New England Journal of Medicine* 342: 1149–1155.

Vermorken, J.B., et al. 1999. "Active Specific Immunotherapy for Stage II and Stage III Human Colon Cancer: A Randomised Trial." *Lancet* 353: 345–50.

Viera, A.J. 1999. "Newer Pharmacologic Alternatives for Erectile Dysfunction." *American Family Physician,* September 15. Online: www.findarticles com.

CHAPTER THIRTEEN: HEALING FROM WITHIN

Alistair, J., et al. 2000. "Association of Involvement in Psychological Self-Regulation with Longer Survival in Patients with Metastatic Cancer: An Exploratory Study." *Advances in Mind–Body Medicine* 16: 276–294.

Johnson, J., et al. 1993. "Role of Support Groups in Cancer Care." *Supportive Care in Cancer* 1: 52–56.

Kramish, C.M., et al. 2001. "Health Behavior Changes After Colon Cancer: A Comparison of Findings from Face-to-Face and On-line Focus Groups." *Family & Community Health* 24: 11–103.

Tache, V., et al. 2001. "Stress and the Gastrointestinal Tract III. Stress-Related Alterations of Gut Motor Function: Role of Brain Corticotropin-Releasing Factor Receptors." *American Journal of Physiology. Gastrointestinal and Liver Physiology* 280: G173–G177.

Index

abdominal resection (APR), 149–50
bowel prep, 145–46
bowel resection, 121
colostomy, 142, 150–51
laparoscopy, 147–48
low anterior resection (LAR), 148
lymph node removal, 121
metastatic cancer and, 151
partial coletomy, 146–47
potential complications, 152–53
preparing for surgery, checklist, 153–54
presurgery tests and evaluation, 144–45
(table)
recovering from, 155–62
recurrent colorectal cancer and, 151–52
state of your health and, 143
subtotal and total colectomy, 147
surgical path report, 121–24
transanal excision, 149
See also recovery from surgery
symptoms of colorectal cancer
abdominal discomfort, 16
anemia, 16, 20
blockage in colon, 20
blood in stool, 15, 20
change in bowel habits, 15
checklist, 16
early stage, absence of, 14, 15, 20
fatigue, 16
iron deficiency, 16
loss of appetite/unexplained weight loss, 15
of recurrence, 210–11

t'ai chi, 196–97
effectiveness, 196
safety, 197
Tartikoff, Lilly, xii, xix
treatment
chemotherapy, 163–73, 174–76
get informed (questions to ask), 139–40
lifestyle changes following, 211–15
radiation, 161–62, 164, 165–66, 173–76
second opinion, 140

surgery, 142–62
treatment log, 141
See also chemotherapy; complementary
therapies; follow-up care; radiation;
surgery
turmeric, 109–10

ulcerative colitis, 95, 147
inflammatory polyp and, 119
ulcers, 6, 56
upper endoscopy, 57

vascular abnormalities, 52
virtual colonoscopy, 62–63
vitamin D, 94, 101–2, 112, 212
in dairy products, 82
dosage, 102, 212
food sources, 102
vitamin E, 94, 104–5, 112
colorectal cancer and, 104
dosage, 104–5
food sources, 104
precautions, 105
Visicol, 43
residue (MCC), 43–44

water
fiber intake and, 77, 83–84
importance, 83–84
recommendation, 84, 213
recovering from surgery and, 156
urine color and, 84
weight
calories daily, maximum, 212
excess and body shape, risk of colorectal
cancer and, 28, 69
Weill Medical College, Cornell University,
125
Winawer, Sidney, 37

yoga, 197
effectiveness, 197
Kripalu form, 197
safety, 197

Colorectal Cancer

EDUCATIONAL CD-ROM

What you need to know

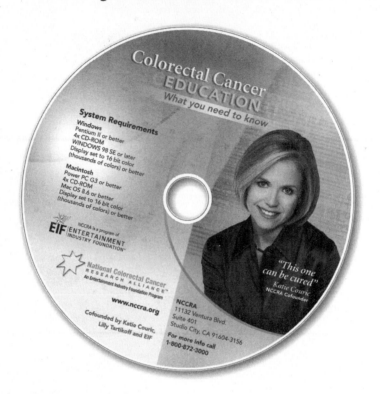

Take charge of your health!

Learn more about the latest tests, treatments and resources available for colorectal cancer. You'll see remarkable videos to better understand how colorectal cancer begins and develops, and how easy it is to be screened.

Visit www.eif.nccra.org or call 1-800-872-3000 to order your FREE CD-ROM from the National Colorectal Cancer Research Alliance (NCCRA), a program of the Entertainment Industry Foundation.

The multimedia CD-ROM was created with help from leading physician groups: American Gastroenterological Association, American College of Obstetricians and Gynecologists, American Society of Colon and Rectal Surgeons, and the Foundation For Digestive Health and Nutrition, as well as NCCRA's Medical Advisory Board.

NCCRA was co-founded in March of 2000 by journalist Katie Couric, cancer activist Lilly Tartikoff, and the Entertainment Industry Foundation. NCCRA is dedicated to the eradication of colorectal cancer by promoting the importance of early medical screening and funding research to develop better tests, treatments and, ultimately, a cure.

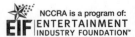

NCCRA is a program of:
EIF ENTERTAINMENT INDUSTRY FOUNDATION™

www.eif.nccra.org | 800.872.3000